# Food & Nutrition

Editor: Tina Brand

Volume 339

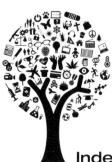

Independence Educational Publishers

First published by Independence Educational Publishers

The Studio, High Green

Great Shelford

Cambridge CB22 5EG

England

## Copyright

## Photocopy licence

ISBN–13: 978 1 86168 790 6

## Printed in Great Britain

Zenith Print Group

# Contents

# Introduction

FOOD & NUTRITION is Volume 339 in the **ISSUES** series. The aim of the series is to offer current, diverse information about important issues in our world, from a UK perspective.

## ABOUT FOOD & NUTRITION

The UK has one of the highest rates of obesity in Europe, and the rate is rising faster than that of the US. So how can we overcome this obesity crisis? Being obese or overweight can lead to many health issues, and in this book we explore how eating a healthy, nutritious diet can help. From five-a-day to planning meal budgets there is advice on how to make healthier choices

## OUR SOURCES

Titles in the **ISSUES** series are designed to function as educational resource books, providing a balanced overview of a specific subject.

The information in our books is comprised of facts, articles and opinions from many different sources, including:

⇨ Newspaper reports and opinion pieces

⇨ Website factsheets

⇨ Magazine and journal articles

⇨ Statistics and surveys

⇨ Government reports

⇨ Literature from special interest groups.

## A NOTE ON CRITICAL EVALUATION

Because the information reprinted here is from a number of different sources, readers should bear in mind the origin of the text and whether the source is likely to have a particular bias when presenting information (or when conducting their research). It is hoped that, as you read about the many aspects of the issues explored in this book, you will critically evaluate the information presented.

It is important that you decide whether you are being presented with facts or opinions. Does the writer give a biased or unbiased report? If an opinion is being expressed, do you agree with the writer? Is there potential bias to the 'facts' or statistics behind an article?

## ASSIGNMENTS

In the back of this book, you will find a selection of assignments designed to help you engage with the articles you have been reading and to explore your own opinions. Some tasks will take longer than others and there is a mixture of design, writing and research-based activities that you can complete alone or in a group.

## Useful weblinks

www.bupa.co.uk/health-information

www.cam.ac.uk

www.cancerresearchuk.org

www.diabetes.co.uk

www.diabetestimes.co.uk

www.eufic.org

www.fareshare.org.uk

www.foodfoundation.org.uk

www.fullfact.org

www.gov.uk

www.imperial.ac.uk

www.independent.co.uk

www.inews.co.uk

www.nhs.uk

www.nuffieldhealth.com

www.nutrition.org.uk

www.telegraph.co.uk

www.theconversation.com

www.thefoodrush.com

www.who.int

www.wolverhampton.gov.uk

## FURTHER RESEARCH

At the end of each article we have listed its source and a website that you can visit if you would like to conduct your own research. Please remember to critically evaluate any sources that you consult and consider whether the information you are viewing is accurate and unbiased.

# Chapter 1

# Obesity Crisis?

# Obesity and overweight

## Key facts

⇨ **Worldwide obesity has nearly tripled since 1975.**

⇨ **In 2016, more than 1.9 billion adults, 18 years and older, were overweight. Of these over 650 million were obese.**

⇨ **39% of adults aged 18 years and over were overweight in 2016, and 13% were obese.**

⇨ **Most of the world's population live in countries where overweight and obesity kills more people than underweight.**

⇨ **41 million children under the age of five were overweight or obese in 2016.**

⇨ **Over 340 million children and adolescents aged five to 19 were overweight or obese in 2016.**

⇨ **Obesity is preventable.**

## What are obesity and overweight?

Overweight and obesity are defined as abnormal or excessive fat accumulation that may impair health.

Body mass index (BMI) is a simple index of weight-for-height that is commonly used to classify overweight and obesity in adults. It is defined as a person's weight in kilograms divided by the square of his height in metres (kg/m²).

### Adults

For adults, WHO defines overweight and obesity as follows:

⇨ overweight is a BMI greater than or equal to 25

⇨ obesity is a BMI greater than or equal to 30.

BMI provides the most useful population-level measure of overweight and obesity as it is the same for both sexes and for all ages of adults. However, it should be considered a rough guide because it may not correspond to the same degree of fatness in different individuals.

For children, age needs to be considered when defining overweight and obesity.

### Children under five years of age

For children under five years of age:

⇨ overweight is weight-for-height greater than two standard deviations above WHO Child Growth Standards median; and

⇨ obesity is weight-for-height greater than three standard deviations above the WHO Child Growth Standards median.

### Children aged between five and 19 years

Overweight and obesity are defined as follows for children aged between 5 and 19 years:

⇨ overweight is BMI-for-age greater than one standard deviation above the WHO Growth Reference median; and

⇨ obesity is greater than two standard deviations above the WHO Growth Reference median.

## Facts about overweight and obesity

Some recent WHO global estimates follow.

⇨ In 2016, more than 1.9 billion adults aged 18 years and older were overweight. Of these over 650 million adults were obese.

⇨ In 2016, 39% of adults aged 18 years and over (39% of men and 40% of women) were overweight.

⇨ Overall, about 13% of the world's adult population (11% of men and 15% of women) were obese in 2016.

⇨ The worldwide prevalence of obesity nearly tripled between 1975 and 2016.

In 2016, an estimated 41 million children under the age of five years were overweight or obese. Once considered a high-income country problem, overweight and obesity are now on the rise in low- and middle-income countries, particularly in urban settings. In Africa, the number of overweight children under five has increased by nearly 50 per cent since 2000. Nearly half of the children under five who were overweight or obese in 2016 lived in Asia.

Over 340 million children and adolescents aged five to 19 were overweight or obese in 2016.

The prevalence of overweight and obesity among children and adolescents aged five to 19 has risen dramatically from just 4% in 1975 to just over 18% in 2016. The rise has occurred similarly among both boys and girls: in 2016, 18% of girls and 19% of boys were overweight.

While just under 1% of children and adolescents aged five to 19 were obese in 1975, more 124 million children and adolescents (6% of girls and 8% of boys) were obese in 2016.

Overweight and obesity are linked to more deaths worldwide than underweight. Globally there are more people who are obese than underweight – this occurs in every region except parts of sub–Saharan Africa and Asia.

## What causes obesity and overweight?

The fundamental cause of obesity and overweight is an energy imbalance between calories consumed and calories expended. Globally, there has been:

⇨ an increased intake of energy-dense foods that are high in fat; and

⇨ an increase in physical inactivity due to the increasingly sedentary nature of many forms of work, changing modes of transportation, and increasing urbanisation.

Changes in dietary and physical activity patterns are often the result of environmental and societal changes associated with development and lack of supportive policies in sectors such as health, agriculture, transport, urban planning, environment, food processing, distribution, marketing and education.

## What are common health consequences of overweight and obesity?

Raised BMI is a major risk factor for noncommunicable diseases such as:

⇨ cardiovascular diseases (mainly heart disease and stroke), which were the leading cause of death in 2012;

⇨ diabetes;

⇨ musculoskeletal disorders (especially osteoarthritis – a highly disabling degenerative disease of the joints);

⇨ some cancers (including endometrial, breast, ovarian, prostate, liver, gallbladder, kidney and colon).

The risk for these noncommunicable diseases increases, with increases in BMI.

Childhood obesity is associated with a higher chance of obesity, premature death and disability in adulthood. But in addition to increased future risks, obese children experience breathing difficulties, increased risk of fractures, hypertension, early markers of cardiovascular disease, insulin resistance and psychological effects.

## Facing a double burden of disease

Many low- and middle-income countries are now facing a 'double burden' of disease.

⇨ While these countries continue to deal with the problems of infectious diseases and undernutrition, they are also experiencing a rapid upsurge in noncommunicable disease risk factors such as obesity and overweight, particularly in urban settings.

⇨ It is not uncommon to find undernutrition and obesity co-existing within the same country, the same community and the same household.

Children in low- and middle-income countries are more vulnerable to inadequate pre-natal, infant and young child nutrition. At the same time, these children are exposed to high-fat, high-sugar, high-salt, energy-dense and micronutrient-poor foods, which tend to be lower in cost but also lower in nutrient quality. These dietary patterns, in conjunction with lower levels of physical activity, result in sharp increases in childhood obesity while undernutrition issues remain unsolved.

## How can overweight and obesity be reduced?

Overweight and obesity, as well as their related noncommunicable diseases, are largely preventable. Supportive environments and communities are fundamental in shaping people's choices, by making the choice of healthier foods and regular physical activity the easiest choice (the choice that is the most accessible, available and affordable), and therefore preventing overweight and obesity.

At the individual level, people can:

⇨ limit energy intake from total fats and sugars;

⇨ increase consumption of fruit and vegetables, as well as legumes, whole grains and nuts; and

⇨ engage in regular physical activity (60 minutes a day for children and 150 minutes spread through the week for adults).

Individual responsibility can only have its full effect where people have access to a healthy lifestyle. Therefore, at the societal level it is important to support individuals in following the recommendations above, through sustained implementation of evidence-based and population-based policies that make regular physical activity and healthier dietary choices available, affordable and easily accessible to everyone, particularly to the poorest individuals. An example of such a policy is a tax on sugar-sweetened beverages.

The food industry can play a significant role in promoting healthy diets by:

⇨ reducing the fat, sugar and salt content of processed foods;

⇨ ensuring that healthy and nutritious choices are available and affordable to all consumers;

⇨ restricting marketing of foods high in sugars, salt and fats, especially those foods aimed at children and teenagers; and

⇨ ensuring the availability of healthy food choices and supporting regular physical activity practice in the workplace.

## WHO response

Adopted by the World Health Assembly in 2004, the *WHO Global Strategy on Diet, Physical Activity and Health* describes the actions needed to support healthy diets and regular physical activity. The Strategy calls upon all stakeholders to take action at global, regional and local levels to improve diets and physical activity patterns at the population level.

'The Political Declaration of the High Level Meeting of the United Nations General Assembly on the Prevention and Control of Non-communicable Diseases' of September 2011, recognises the critical importance of reducing unhealthy diet and physical inactivity. The political declaration commits to advancing the implementation of the 'WHO Global Strategy on Diet, Physical Activity and Health', including, where appropriate, through the introduction of policies and actions aimed at promoting healthy diets and increasing physical activity in the entire population.

WHO has also developed the Global Action Plan for the Prevention and Control of Noncommunicable Diseases 2013–2020' which aims to achieve the commitments of the UN Political Declaration on Noncommunicable diseases (NCDs) which was endorsed by Heads of State and Government in September 2011. The 'Global Action Plan' will contribute to progress on nine global NCD targets to be attained by 2025, including a 25% relative reduction in premature mortality from NCDs by 2025 and a halt in the rise of global obesity to match the rates of 2010.

The World Health Assembly welcomed the report of the Commission on Ending Childhood Obesity (2016) and its six recommendations to address the obesogenic environment and critical periods in the life course to tackle childhood obesity. The implementation plan to guide countries in taking action to implement the recommendations of the Commission was welcomed by the World Health Assembly in 2017.

*16 February 2018*

⇨ The above information is reprinted with kind permission from World Health Organization. Please visit www.who.int for further information.

# UK named most overweight nation in Western Europe as obesity rate rises faster than US

**Around 27 per cent of Britons are now clinically obese, and another 36 per cent are overweight.**

*By Lizzie Dearden, Home Affairs Correspondent*

The UK is the most overweight nation in Western Europe, with levels of obesity growing faster than in the US, a new report has warned.

The Organisation for Economic Cooperation and Development (OECD) said Britain was the sixth-worst country in its 35 member states, coming behind Mexico, the USA, New Zealand, Finland and Australia.

Around 27 per cent of the population are now clinically obese and another 36 per cent are overweight, making the combined figure among the highest in the world.

'Obesity has risen sharply since 1990, when it affected only 14 per cent of adults,' said the OECD's annual *Health at a Glance* report.

'The overall health of British people is similar to the OECD average, considering life expectancy and other general measures of health status… but obesity rates are considerably worse.'

It listed the UK as among countries with 'historically high' rates, but said it was also the country where obesity was rising the fastest – increasing by 92 per cent, compared to 65 per cent in the US.

'Obesity means higher risk of chronic illnesses, particularly hypertension, cholesterol, diabetes and cardiovascular diseases,' the report added, saying that NHS campaigns were attempting to tackle the causes of obesity but 'much more can still be done'.

Other concerns highlighted by the OECD including alcohol consumption among teenagers in the UK, where almost a third of 15-year-olds say they have been drunk at least twice in their life – far above the OECD average of 22 per cent.

For adults, smoking rates and the amount of alcohol consumed by the average person is falling.

The research used the World Health Organization's definition of obesity as a BMI of 30 and above, and of overweight between 25 and 30.

It came after NHS England ordered hospitals to take 'super-size' chocolate bars and bags of sweet snacks off shelves.

Last month it announced a 250-calorie limit on confectionery sold in hospital canteens, shops, vending machines and other outlets to help fight obesity, diabetes and tooth decay.

Simon Stevens, NHS England's chief executive, said: 'The NHS is now stepping up action to combat the 'super-size' snack culture which is causing an epidemic of obesity, preventable diabetes, tooth decay, heart disease and cancer.'

Soft drinks will also be hit by the Government's new 'sugar tax' when it comes into effect in April 2018.

Tax on drinks with more than five grams of sugar per 100ml will be levied by 18p per litre, while those with eight grams or more of sugar per 100ml will have an extra tax of 24p per litre.

While generating revenue, proponents hope the move will also force brands to reformulate their drinks to reduce sugar content and avoid penalties.

*11 November 2017*

⇨ The above information is reprinted with kind permission from *The Independent*. Please visit www.independent.co.uk for further information.

# Millennials top obesity chart before reaching middle age

**M**ore than seven in ten millennials – those born between the early 80s and mid-90s – are set to be overweight or obese between the ages of 35–44, according to estimates by Cancer Research UK.

This compares to around five in ten baby boomers – those born between 1945–55 – who were overweight or obese at the same age.

This means millennials are the most overweight generation since current records began.

Being overweight or obese as an adult is linked to 13 different types of cancer including breast, bowel and kidney cancer, but only 15% of people in the UK are aware of the link.

> *"Being overweight is the UK's biggest preventable cause of cancer after smoking, but most people don't know about this substantial risk. If more people become aware of the link it may help spare not just millennials, but all generations from cancer."*
> *– Alison Cox, Cancer Research UK*

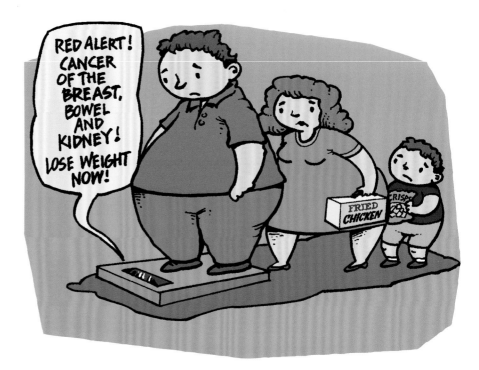

Cancer Research UK has launched a UK-wide campaign to increase awareness that obesity is a cause of cancer.

Alison Cox, Cancer Research UK's director of prevention, said: 'Being overweight is the UK's biggest preventable cause of cancer after smoking, but most people don't know about this substantial risk. If more people become aware of the link it may help spare not just millennials, but all generations from cancer.

'The Government must play a part to help people make healthy food choices. We're campaigning for a ban on junk food adverts before the 9pm watershed to protect young people from advertising tactics which all too often promote fattening foods.'

Professor Linda Bauld, Cancer Research UK's prevention expert, said: 'Research shows that our evolving environment has a vital role to play in the obesity crisis. Clever marketing tactics by the food industry and greater access to unhealthy food are all likely to have contributed to the rise in obesity rates.

'Extra body fat doesn't just sit there; it sends messages around the body that can cause damage to cells. This damage can build up over time and increase the risk of cancer in the same way that damage from smoking causes cancer.

'While these estimates sound bleak, we can stop them becoming a reality. Millennials are known for following seemingly healthy food trends, but nothing beats a balanced diet. Eating plenty of fruit, vegetables and other fibre-filled foods like wholegrains, and cutting down on junk food is the best way to keep a healthy weight.'

Cancer Research UK's campaign will launch across the UK on posters, radio, social and digital media.

To highlight the link, the charity handed out fake cigarette packets to shoppers in Aylesbury posing the question: What is the second biggest preventable cause of cancer? Shoppers got a big surprise on discovering the packs contained chips, and the answer was obesity.

Lottie Goodchild, 24, of Aylesbury said: 'It's shocking, but not surprising. It's important people know about the link because so many in this country, including the younger generation, are practically obese without even knowing it.

'We need families to support each other to keep a healthy balanced lifestyle, and we need the Government to provide the best possible environment for this to happen.'

*26 February 2018*

⇨ The above information is reprinted with kind permission from Cancer Research UK. Please visit www.cancerresearchuk.org for further information.

# Shoppers eat an extra 17,000 calories a year because of 'supersize' tactics

*By Laura Donnelly, Health Editor*

Supersize tactics by retailers mean the average person is consuming an extra 17,000 calories a year – which could mean five pounds weight gain – health experts have warned.

The Royal Society of Public Health said consumers are facing more than 100 attempts each year by shops and fast-food chains to 'up-sell' unhealthy foods and drinks each year.

The charity said soaring obesity levels were being fuelled by pushy sales assistants, trained to ask customers if they wanted to 'go large', upgrade to a meal deal, or add cut-price chocolate to their purchase.

It urged retailers to stop linking staff pay to the success of efforts to pressure customers into buying more junk food.

The report carried out with Slimming World, found that over the course of a week, 'verbal pushes' meant 34 per cent of customers ended up buying a larger coffee than requested, with 33 per cent upgrading to meal deals, and 36 per cent adding chocolate to their shop.

The report, from a survey of more than 2,000 UK adults, found that consumers face an average of 106 verbal pushes annually, which led to an extra 330 calories a week, or 17,000 calories a year.

The extra calories could mean a potential weight gain of five pounds, the report said.

> **Young people aged 18 to 24 are the most likely to experience up-selling, with the study finding that they consume an extra 750 calories a week as a result, which could mean an annual gain of up to 11 pounds.**

The charity urged businesses to pledge to only up-sell healthy food and drink, and said shops should stop paying staff commission for hitting 'up-selling' targets.

The research found that those who were persuaded to supersize on average spent 17 per cent more for 55 per cent more calories, with special offers reserved for the least healthy fare.

RSPH chief executive Shirley Cramer said: 'Obesity is the public health challenge of our generation and if not addressed urgently could tip over the point of no return.

'Almost everyone can relate to the feeling of being pressured into buying extra calories through up-selling.'

The charity and diet company are urging consumers to use the hashtag #JustThisThanks to fight back against the trend, which the head of the NHS has previously described as 'a form of health pollution.'

*7 September 2017*

⇨ The above information is reprinted with kind permission from *The Telegraph*. Please visit www.telegraph.co.uk for further information.

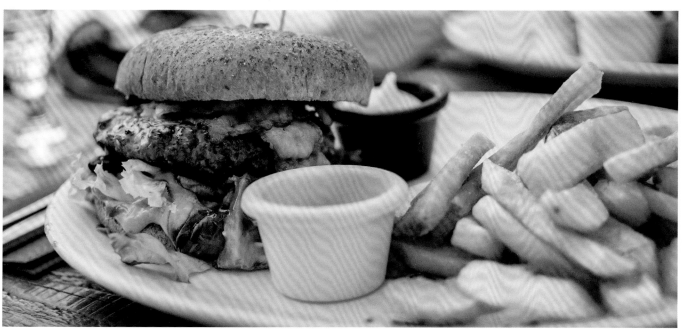

# 28% of two to 15-year-olds in England estimated to be overweight or obese

## Claim

Almost a third of children aged two to 15 are overweight or obese.

## Conclusion

An NHS survey estimates that 28% of children aged two to 15 in England were overweight or obese in 2016.

> **'Data shows that almost a third of children aged two to 15 are overweight or obese.'**
>
> **The Guardian,** 23 April 2018

In England, an estimated 16% of children aged two to 15 were obese in 2016, and a further 12% were overweight (but not obese). That means 28% of two to 15-year-olds were overweight or obese – so just over a quarter.

29% of girls were estimated to be overweight or obese, and 26% of boys were.

Being overweight or obese is defined in terms of body mass index (BMI) – essentially weight divided by height. A child's BMI is measured against a reference chart of BMI levels from 1990. A child whose BMI is in the top 5% of that chart is considered obese, and those in the next 10% down are considered overweight.

The NHS says BMI 'is a good way of finding out whether a child is a healthy weight' but also that 'The BMI can't tell the difference between excess fat, muscle, or bone.' They say it is 'a straightforward and convenient method of assessing someone's weight' and can be used as 'a starting point for further discussion with your GP about your weight and your general health.'

The issue is more prevalent among older children. 23% of those aged two to 10 were overweight or obese, compared to 36% of those aged 11–15.

These figures are estimates, based on a survey of adults and children in England, and should not be treated as exact.

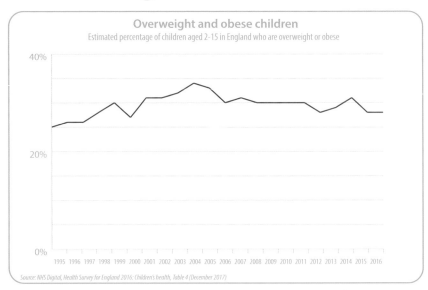

**Overweight and obese children**
Estimated percentage of children aged 2-15 in England who are overweight or obese

Source: NHS Digital, Health Survey for England 2016: Children's health, Table 4 (December 2017)

The estimated level of overweight or obese children has remained quite stable in recent years. Levels were highest in the mid-2000s, and since 2006 they have fluctuated between 28% and 31%.

## There are other assessments of obesity

The National Childhood Measurement Programme (NCMP) is another assessment of childhood obesity, focusing on children at two specific age points: children in Reception, aged four to five, and in Year 6, aged ten to 11.

It finds that 23% of children aged four to five in England were overweight or obese in 2016/17, and 34% of children aged ten to 11 were. These figures use the same definitions of overweight and obese, and give a similar impression to the data looked at above.

Because it's based on a larger sample size, and focuses on two specific age points, the NCMP data allows for more detailed assessments. The House of Commons Library reports that, based on the NCMP data, 'children in the most deprived areas are around twice as likely to be obese' as those in the least deprived areas, both at age four to five, and ten to 11.

The most and least deprived areas are defined those in the top and bottom 10% in terms of the 2015 Index of Multiple Deprivation, published by the (then) Department for Communities and Local Government.

## The rest of the UK

In Wales, an estimated 27% of children aged four to five were overweight or obese in 2016/17, based on the Childhood Measurement Programme for Wales.

In Scotland, an estimated 23% of four to five-year-olds were 'at risk' of being overweight or obese in 2016/17. Scotland measures children as overweight or obese in the same way as England and Wales, but terms them 'at risk'.

In Northern Ireland, an estimated 23% of two to ten-year-olds and 29% of 11–15-year-olds were obese or overweight in 2016/17. But this is a very uncertain figure. It's based on a relatively small sample size, meaning the actual figures could be significantly higher or lower. In the last few years, around a quarter of children aged two to ten have been estimated as overweight or obese, and a similar proportion of 11–15-year-olds have been as well.

*23 April 2018*

⇨ The above information is reprinted with kind permission from Full Fact. Please visit www.fullfact.org for further information.

# Soft Drinks Industry Levy comes into effect

## The 'Sugar Tax' will help to reduce sugar in soft drinks and tackle childhood obesity.

From Friday (6 April 2018), millions of children across the UK will benefit from the Government's key milestone in tackling childhood obesity, as the Soft Drinks Industry Levy comes into effect.

The tax on soft drinks, commonly referred to as the 'Sugar Tax', has already resulted in over 50% of manufacturers reducing the sugar content of drinks since it was announced in March 2016 – the equivalent of 45 million kg of sugar every year.

Soft drinks manufacturers who don't reformulate will pay the levy, which is expected to raise £240 million each year. This money will go towards doubling the Primary Sports Premium, the creation of a Healthy Pupils Capital Fund to help schools upgrade their sports facilities, and give children access to top quality PE equipment.

The levy will also give a funding boost for healthy school breakfast clubs.

Exchequer Secretary to the Treasury, Robert Jenrick MP visited the Lucozade Ribena Suntory factory today (5 April 2018), which has led the way in reformulating its drinks alongside the likes of Tesco and Irn Bru.

He commented:

*'The Soft Drinks Levy is one part of our plan to tackle childhood obesity. From Friday, soft drinks which contain too much added sugar will need to pay a fee.'*

*'All revenues raised through the levy will directly fund new sports facilities in schools as well as healthy breakfast clubs, ensuring children lead healthier lives.*

*'We want to persuade manufacturers to reformulate their drinks and lower the sugar content. In the time between announcing this policy and it taking effect today, more than half of all soft drinks have been reformulated to lower the sugar content, including many of the best known soft drinks. We hope that will continue in the months and years to come.'*

In England alone, a third of children are obese or overweight when they leave primary school, and evidence shows that 80% of kids who are obese in their early teens will go on to be obese adults.

Public Health Minister, Steve Brine MP remarked:

*'Our teenagers consume nearly a bathtub of sugary drinks each year on average, fuelling a worrying obesity trend in this country. The Soft Drinks Industry Levy is ground-breaking policy that will help to reduce sugar intake, whilst funding sports programmes and nutritious breakfast clubs for children.'*

*'The progress made so far on our obesity plan is promising – but with one in three children still leaving primary school*

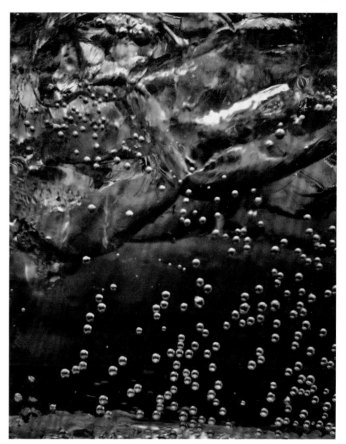

*overweight or obese, we have not ruled out doing more in future.'*

*Notes*

⇨ The aim of the Soft Drinks Industry Levy is to encourage companies to reformulate their soft drinks. Since the levy was announced two years ago, the expected amount of revenue has gone down from £520 million in Year 1 to £240 million. Even before coming into effect, the levy is already working – over 50% of manufacturers have reformulated their drinks

⇨ Even if revenue from the levy declines, funding for schools and children will stay the same

⇨ The rates companies will need to pay are as follows:

· 24p per litre of drink if it contains eight grams of sugar per 100 millilitres

· 18p per litre of drink if it contains between five to eight grams of sugar per 100 millilitres

*5 April 2018*

⇨ The above information is reprinted with kind permission from HM Treasury. Please visit www.gov.uk for further information.

# Sugar tax: what you need to know

**An article from** The Conversation.

THE C**O**NVERSATION

*By Professor Corinna Hawkes, Centre for Food Policy, Department of Sociology*

If you like swigging sugary drinks, you might get a bit of a surprise next time you go to buy one, as a so–called sugar tax has now come into force in the UK.

From now on, drinks with a sugar content of more than 5g per 100ml will be taxed 18p per litre and 24p for drinks with 8g or more. It's hoped the tax will help to reduce sugar intake, as scientists have shown that sugary drinks lead to weight gain and diabetes. Figures show that 58 per cent of women, 68 per cent of men and 34 per cent of ten- to 11-year-olds in the UK are classed as overweight or obese.

Of course, a tax alone is not going to solve the obesity problem overnight. Sugary drinks may be a leading source of sugar in the UK diet, but they are not the only contributor to obesity. So while we are not going to see obesity prevalence crashing down anytime soon, what taxes can do is contribute to change.

## How to reduce sugar

The UK sugar tax aims to incentivise sugar reduction in drinks. Because it is imposed on drinks over a certain sugar threshold, manufacturers have the option of lowering sugar levels to avoid the tax. This way, the Government is sending a clear message to the industry: get your act together and get sugar down.

On this measure of success, we don't have to wait for the tax to be implemented to know that it has had an effect. According to the UK Treasury, over 50 per cent of soft drinks manufacturers (including retailer own-brands) have already reduced sugar levels, responding to the stick of legislation. So much so, in fact, that the Treasury has downgraded its forecast of how much money the levy will bring in – still standing at an impressive £240 million.

The taxes will also make a contribution to the funding of programmes designed to reduce obesity. Such 'earmarking' of taxes is relatively rare, but in the UK the tax was introduced in the March 2016 budget with the explicit goal to 'fund a doubling of the primary schools sports premium'.

We know this approach is workable. In 2015, Jamie Oliver voluntarily imposed a 10p extra charge on the sugary drinks served in his restaurants, encouraging others to do the same. The proceeds were donated to The Children's Health Fund. In the two- and-a-half years since, the fund has given away £162,000 in grants to improve child health. And according to Sustain – the NGO that manages the fund – 146,000 children have benefited from improved access to drinking water, as a result of the extra charge.

## Will it change what people buy?

The UK Government has not made changing people's dietary habits an explicit aim of the tax. But evidence from elsewhere does suggest people buy less when a tax comes into force. For example, in Mexico – which introduced a one peso per litre excise tax on sugary drinks in 2014 – purchases of taxed drinks fell by almost eight per cent in the following two years. Larger decreases were seen in households at the lowest socioeconomic level. And people also bought more of the untaxed drinks – notably water.

In the Mexico case, however, we don't actually know if people started buying fewer sugary drinks because of the price hike, or because of another reason. This is because the data simply measures the decline after the tax, not why the decline is happening. So while prices are likely to have a played a role, there could be another mechanism at work. It could be, for example, that the tax started a conversation, raised awareness, got the industry talking about what it would do in response, and stimulated other actions to reduce consumption.

## The lasting measure of success

Getting people talking, even arguing, about the tax is also an important part in all of this. Is it fair, as it affects people who are poor more than the rich? Why do we need what is essentially a punitive measure to get industry to act? If we are against the idea, then what else would work better and can we prove it?

These questions are important because it's when these conversations percolate through society, that norms can change. Less so-called nanny statism and more people working it out for themselves. Working out, perhaps, that producing and consuming a lot of sugary drinks is not normal at all, but something weird that should be relegated to the past.

An important measure of the success of the Soft Drinks Industry Levy, then, will be if it contributes to changing these norms – in industry and society. And if it does, it will help to contribute towards a healthier society and healthier people.

*6 April 2018*

⇨ The above information is reprinted with kind permission from *The Conversation*. Please visit www. theconversation.com for further information.

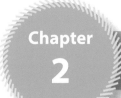
# How the war changed nutrition: from there to now

Nutrition knowledge today owes much to the work done during the war. From food survey to food rationing we learnt valuable lessons regarding nutritional requirements and how these could be provided to everyone in the population at a time when many foods were scarce.

## Key nutrition dates

*1940*

National Food Survey established

*1941*

Nutritional standards for school meals introduced

*1942*

Mandatory fortification of margarine with vitamins A and D began

*1944*

First Food Labelling Order

*1944*

First Proceedings of the Nutrition Society published

## Ministry of Food (1939–1955)

The Ministry of Food was set up in 1939 to deal with the problem of providing a nutritionally adequate diet for people in Great Britain during the Second World War. It played an important role, being the first organisation responsible for a nutrition policy in the UK. The Ministry controlled all food supplies, food reserve stocks and distribution, and had local and regional committees to give expert information and organise the use of gardens, waste land and allotments for producing food locally. The Ministry became a permanent Department of State in 1946 until 1955, when it was subsumed within the Department for Agriculture and Fisheries to become the Ministry of Agriculture, Fisheries and Food (MAFF), which was formally dissolved in 2002, and its responsibilities were split between the Department for Environment, Food and Rural Affairs (Defra) and Food Standards Agency (FSA).

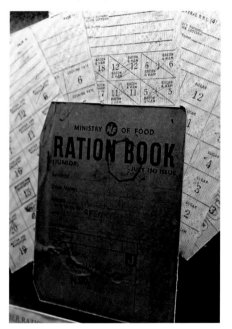

## National Food Survey (NFS)

The NFS (now known as the Family Food Survey) is the longest-running continuous survey of household food consumption and expenditure in the world. It was originally set up in 1940 by the then Ministry of Food to monitor the adequacy of the diet of urban 'working class' households in wartime, but it was extended in 1950 to become representative of households in wartime, throughout Great Britain. It provides a wealth of information that has made a major contribution to the study of the changing patterns of household food consumption.

## Rationing

During the Second World War, the British Government introduced food rationing to make sure that everyone received their fair share of the limited food that was available Food rationing started in 1940 and finally ended in 1954. A system of food rationing to ensure fair distribution of available food. To ensure good health, the amounts of available foods to cover people's nutrient needs were calculated by scientists and statisticians. The wartime food shortages forced people to adopt new eating patterns. Most people ate less meat, fat, eggs and sugar than they had eaten before, but people who had previously consumed a poor diet were able to increase their intake of protein and vitamins because they received the same ration as everybody else. Thus, many people consumed a better diet during wartime food rationing than before the war years and this had a marked effect on health outcomes; infant mortality rates declined, and the average age at which people died from natural causes increased.

⇨ The above information is reprinted with kind permission from British Nutrition Foundation. Please visit www.nutrition.org.uk for further information.

# Where are consumers getting their nutrition information from?

*By Dr Stacey Lockyer, Nutrition Scientist*

Data from the National Diet and Nutrition Survey shows that as a nation we aren't meeting the vast majority of dietary guidelines. Our intake of saturated fat, free sugars and salt are too high and we are not getting enough fibre, fruit and vegetables, and oily fish. Two-thirds of adults are overweight and obese and there is also evidence of inadequate micronutrient intake. So do consumers have an accurate understanding of what a healthy diet is, and where are they getting their information from?

In a national survey, equal proportions of consumers believed that food labels and the Internet were the most reliable sources of information about food. While information on food labels must be accurate by law, health information on the web isn't always correct, which is a concern. However, there is an easy way to check. The Information Standard accreditation scheme, supported by NHS England, is a quality mark which identifies reliable and trustworthy health and social care information so is useful to look out for when looking for nutrition information. The NHS Choices website and around 220 other health organisations including BNF (nutrition.org.uk) are members of the scheme, with the Information Standard logo being displayed on pages providing information for consumers.

Nutritionists, dietitians and health professionals were believed to be the most reliable source by the largest proportion of consumers in the survey. Registered dietitians are qualified health professionals that assess, diagnose and treat diet and nutrition problems at an individual and wider public health level. But perhaps surprisingly, the title 'nutritionist' is not protected by law and so anyone (qualified or unqualified) can call themselves a nutritionist and provide dietary advice which may not be evidence-based. The Association for Nutrition is attempting to tackle this issue with the UK Voluntary Register of Nutritionists. Registrants must demonstrate knowledge and understanding of core competencies in nutrition science and consumers can search for individuals on the register before deciding whether or not to engage with them.

The sudden popularity (or unpopularity) of particular products demonstrates the influence of food bloggers on consumer food choice, and the inclusion or exclusion of these foods may not actually be healthy. For example, coconut oil, heralded as a cure-all product, has a very high saturated fat content, raises blood cholesterol in human studies and there is very little evidence it confers any health benefits. Similarly, honeys, syrups (such as agave and date) and nectars (such as coconut blossom nectar), are often portrayed as healthier choices than table sugar but in fact all count as free sugars, the type of sugars that PHE advise we should minimise in our diets to reduce the risk of both dental caries and weight gain. Fruit juice is a good source of vitamins and smoothies also provide fibre. These count as up to one of your five a day but portions should be limited to 150 ml per day due to their free sugars content, so hold off juicing everything in the fridge!

The concept of 'superfoods' is also misleading. For example, all fruits and vegetables are good for us and eating plenty and a variety is key, not choosing those with the most marketed health halos and a matching high price tag – because a healthy, balanced diet can comprise inexpensive, everyday foods. Finally, avoiding entire food groups such as dairy products or starchy carbohydrates when there is no medical reason to do so is not advisable as this can result in nutritional imbalance and even deficiencies.

UK dietary guidelines are based on the best scientific evidence available so to ensure you are getting all the nutrients you need and reduce your risk of developing chronic diseases, consume a diet that's in line with the Eatwell Guide and importantly, seek dietary information from reputable sources.

*15 June 2017*

⇨ The above information is reprinted with kind permission from British Nutrition Foundation. Please visit www.nutrition.org.uk for further information.

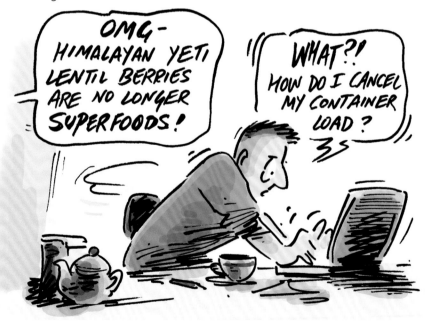

# Eating a balanced diet

***Eating a healthy, balanced diet is an important part of maintaining good health, and can help you feel your best.***

This means eating a wide variety of foods in the right proportions, and consuming the right amount of food and drink to achieve and maintain a healthy body weight.

## Food groups in our diet

The Eatwell Guide shows that to have a healthy, balanced diet, people should try to:

⇨ eat 5 A Day

⇨ base meals on starchy foods like potatoes, bread, rice or pasta

⇨ have some dairy or dairy alternatives (such as soya drinks)

⇨ eat some beans, pulses, fish, eggs, meat and other protein

⇨ choose unsaturated oils and spreads, eaten in small amounts

⇨ drink plenty of fluids.

If you're having foods and drinks that are high in fat, salt and sugar, have these less often and in small amounts.

Try to choose a variety of different foods from the 5 main food groups.

Most people in the UK eat and drink too many calories, too much fat, sugar and salt, and not enough fruit, vegetables, oily fish or fibre.

## Fruit and vegetables: are you getting your 5 A Day?

Fruit and vegetables are a vital source of vitamins and minerals, and should make up just over a third of the food we eat each day.

It's advised that we eat at least 5 portions of a variety of fruit and vegetables every day.

There's evidence that people who eat at least 5 portions a day have a lower risk of heart disease, stroke and some cancers.

Eating 5 portions is not as hard as it sounds. Just one apple, banana, pear or similar-sized fruit is 1 portion (80g).

A slice of pineapple or melon is 1 portion. Three heaped tablespoons of vegetables is another portion.

Having a sliced banana with your morning cereal is a quick way to get 1 portion. Swap your mid-morning biscuit for a tangerine, and add a side salad to your lunch.

Have a portion of vegetables with dinner, and snack on fresh fruit with natural plain yoghurt in the evening to reach your 5 A Day.

## Starchy foods in your diet

Starchy foods should make up just over a third of everything we eat. This means we should base our meals on these foods.

Potatoes with the skins on are a great source of fibre and vitamins. For example, when having boiled potatoes or a jacket potato, eat the skin too.

Try to choose wholegrain or wholemeal varieties of starchy foods, such as brown rice, wholewheat pasta and brown, wholemeal or higher fibre white bread.

They contain more fibre, and usually more vitamins and minerals, than white varieties.

## Milk and dairy foods: go for lower-fat varieties

Milk and dairy foods such as cheese and yoghurt are good sources of protein. They also contain calcium, which helps keep your bones healthy.

To enjoy the health benefits of dairy without eating too much fat, use semi-skimmed, 1% fat or skimmed milk, as well as lower-fat hard cheeses or cottage cheese, and lower-fat, lower-sugar yoghurt.

Unsweetened calcium-fortified dairy alternatives like soya milks, soya yoghurts and soya cheeses also count as part of this food group and can make good alternatives to dairy products.

## Beans, pulses, fish, eggs, meat and other proteins

These foods are all good sources of protein, which is essential for the body to grow and repair itself. They're also good sources of a range of vitamins and minerals.

Meat is a good source of protein, vitamins and minerals, including iron, zinc and B vitamins. It's also one of the main sources of vitamin B12.

Try to eat lean cuts of meat and skinless poultry whenever possible to

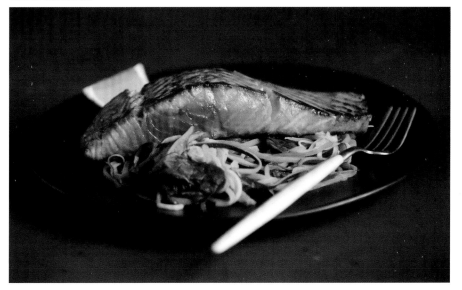

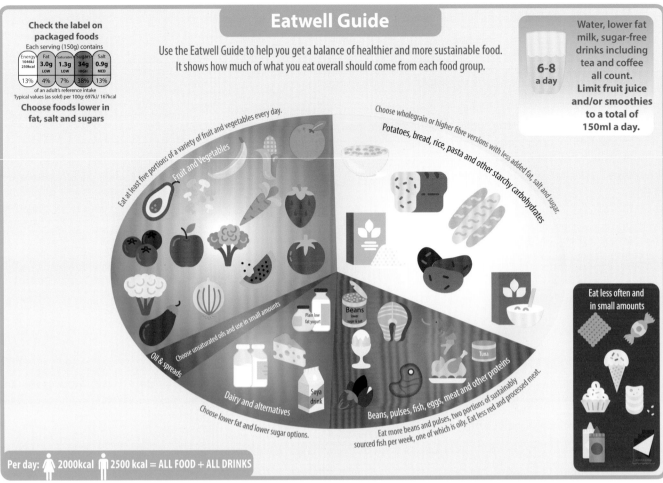

# Eatwell Guide

Use the Eatwell Guide to help you get a balance of healthier and more sustainable food.
It shows how much of what you eat overall should come from each food group.

**Check the label on packaged foods**

Each serving (150g) contains

| Energy 1046kJ 250kcal | Fat 3.0g LOW | Saturates 1.3g LOW | Sugars 34g HIGH | Salt 0.9g MED |
|---|---|---|---|---|
| 13% | 4% | 7% | 38% | 13% |

of an adult's reference intake
Typical values (as sold) per 100g: 697kJ/ 167kcal

**Choose foods lower in fat, salt and sugars**

Eat at least five portions of a variety of fruit and vegetables every day.

**Fruit and Vegetables**

Choose wholegrain or higher fibre versions with less added fat, salt and sugar

**Potatoes, bread, rice, pasta and other starchy carbohydrates**

Water, lower fat milk, sugar-free drinks including tea and coffee all count.
**6-8 a day**
**Limit fruit juice and/or smoothies to a total of 150ml a day.**

**Oil & spreads**
Choose unsaturated oils and use in small amounts

Plain low fat yogurt

Beans lower sugar & salt

Soya drink

**Dairy and alternatives**
Choose lower fat and lower sugar options.

Tuna

**Beans, pulses, fish, eggs, meat and other proteins**
Eat more beans and pulses, two portions of sustainably sourced fish per week, one of which is oily. Eat less red and processed meat.

**Eat less often and in small amounts**

**Per day:** 👩 2000kcal 👨 2500 kcal = ALL FOOD + ALL DRINKS

Source: Public Health England in association with the Welsh Government, Food Standards Scotland and the Food Standards Agency in Northern Ireland

cut down on fat. Always cook meat thoroughly.

Fish is another important source of protein, and contains many vitamins and minerals. Oily fish is particularly rich in omega-3 fatty acids.

Aim for at least 2 portions of fish a week, including 1 portion of oily fish.

You can choose from fresh, frozen or canned, but remember that canned and smoked fish can often be high in salt.

Eggs and pulses (including beans, nuts and seeds) are also great sources of protein.

Nuts are high in fibre and a good alternative to snacks high in saturated fat, but they do still contain high levels of fat, so eat them in moderation.

## Oils and spreads

Some fat in the diet is essential, but should be limited to small amounts.

It's important to get most of our fat from unsaturated oils and spreads.

Swapping to unsaturated fats can help lower cholesterol.

## Eat less saturated fat and sugar

Too much saturated fat can increase the amount of cholesterol in the blood, which increases your risk of developing heart disease, while regularly consuming foods and drinks high in sugar increases your risk of obesity and tooth decay.

*16 March 2016*

⇨ The above information is reproduced with kind permission from the NHS. Please visit www.nhs.uk for further information.

*© Crown Copyright 2018*

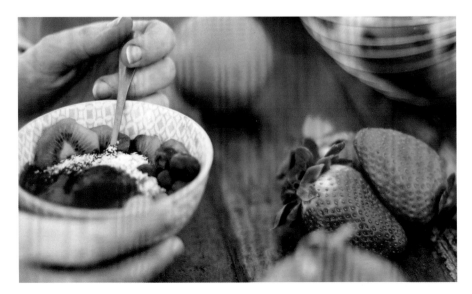

# 3.7 million children in the UK live in households for whom a healthy diet is increasingly unaffordable

⇨ Comparing the estimated cost of Public Health England's (PHE) 'Eatwell Guide' with household income, shows that the bottom 20% of families would have to spend 42% of their after-housing income on food to eat the Government's recommended diet.

⇨ This is nearly four times what the richest 20% of UK families would need to spend on food to meet PHE's Eatwell Guide.

⇨ 3.7 million children in the UK are living in these households, earning less than £15,860, and are likely to be unable to afford a healthy diet as defined by the Government.

⇨ 14 million households (half of all households in the UK) currently don't spend enough to meet the cost of Government's recommended the Eatwell Guide.

⇨ Widening inequality is leading to higher rates of childhood obesity in deprived areas with 26% of children in Year 6 being obese compared to 11% in England's richest communities.

⇨ Findings strengthen calls for a national measurement of food insecurity and the need for further investigation into children's access to healthy food in the UK (led by the Children's Future Food Inquiry)

Wednesday 5 September – New analysis *Affordability of the UK's Eatwell Guide* from independent think tank the The Food Foundation finds that around 3.7 million children in the UK are part of families who earn less than £15,860 and would have to spend 42% of their after-housing income on food to meet the costs of the Government's nutrition guidelines, making a healthy diet most likely unaffordable.

Comparing the estimated cost of the PHE Eatwell Guide (PHE's official guidance on what constitutes a healthy diet and which is based on the latest scientific evidence) to household income in England, Scotland, Northern Ireland and Wales shows that the poorest half of households would need to spend nearly 30% of their after-housing income on food to eat the Government's recommended diet, compared with 12% for the richest half of households.

This analysis comes as children in the UK return to school amid growing concerns over holiday hunger. The availability of free school meals during term-time will be a relief for parents who struggled to feed their children over the holidays.

The unaffordability of a healthy diet for low-income households is highlighted by higher rates of childhood obesity in deprived areas of the country. Over a quarter (26%) of Year 6 children in the most deprived areas of England are obese, but obesity affects just 11% in England's richest communities – and the gap is growing.

The Food Foundation's food affordability research comes as the Children's Future Food Inquiry is gathering evidence from those who have witnessed or experienced children's food insecurity in the UK. With an estimated 3.7 million children living in households that likely cannot afford a healthy diet and record levels of childhood obesity, the parliamentary inquiry is joining calls for a national measurement for food insecurity and next year will present recommendations to policy makers for understanding and tackling children's food insecurity and its consequences in the UK.

## Case study – Elaine from Thanet

Elaine is a mother of four kids who all still live at home. Her husband had to quit work due to ill health and they have recently had their benefits cut by £95 per week. She struggles to balance the weekly budget and estimates she has between £50–60 per week to spend on food. She often finds that it's the least healthy options that are available within her budget.

*'I really try and my kids eat well. But what we are eating is not how I would really like them to eat.'*

*She will be looking for work in September when her youngest child goes back to school but is worried about finding something that will fit around school hours. Currently all her kids receive free school meals and she is concerned that working could also affect that.*

*'I would never let my children go without, but I do go without. I have no social life unless it is something free. Can't afford to go out for a coffee'.*

**Sharon Hodgson MP, Chair of the Children's Future Food Inquiry committee said:**

'It has always been a great concern to me that so many children and families in the UK are at risk of going hungry, or going without a healthy meal each day. That is why I have campaigned for many years to change this, and why I am proud to chair the Children's Future Food Inquiry committee, which is looking into this incredibly important issue.

'It cannot be right that 50% of households in the UK currently have insufficient food budgets to meet the Government's recommended Eatwell Guide. A healthy diet, which we know is important for our health and development, should not be unaffordable to so many people.

'I hope that the Government will look into this issue as a matter of urgency, in order to make eating a healthy diet more affordable.'

**Anna Taylor, Executive Director of the Food Foundation, said:**

'The Government's measurement of household income highlights the fact that millions of families in the UK cannot afford to eat in line with the Government's own dietary guidance. It's crucial that a coordinated cross-government effort develops policy that accounts for the cost of its recommended diet, and creates a food system that does not consign those on lower incomes to the risk of diet–related illness.

'If you or children you know have struggled to access enough food or nutritious diets, share your stories with the Children's Future Food Inquiry evidence portal. The Inquiry is investigating children's food insecurity in the UK, and was launched to hear directly from children and young people about their experiences.'

**Inquiry website:** https://foodfoundation.org.uk/childrens-future-food-inquiry/

**Inquiry portal:** http://www.leedsbeckett.ac.uk/carnegie-school-of-education/child-food-insecurity/

**Twitter:** @CFFinquiry

*September 2018*

⇨ The above information is reprinted with kind permission from The Food Foundation. Please visit www.foodfoundation.org.uk for further information.

*© Food Foundation 2018*

# Criticism over Eatwell Plate amid calls for low-carb approach

**The Eatwell Plate has been slammed in the European Parliament, with the concept of basing diets on starchy foods being branded 'misguided'.**

The guideline says meals should include potatoes, bread, rice, pasta or other starchy carbohydrates, with low or reduced–fat cheese and yoghurt and preferably unsaturated oils and spreads.

It was first published in 1983, with the latest version released by Public Health England and officially known as the Eatwell Guide. According to gov.uk, it is a 'policy tool used to define government recommendations on eating healthily and achieving a balanced diet'.

But cardiologist Dr Aseem Malhotra, the Queen's former doctor Sir Richard Thompson and nutritionist Sarah Macklin, called for an overhaul of official guidelines, advocating a low–carbohydrate, Mediterranean diet to help prevent type 2 diabetes during the debate about public health in Brussels.

Dr Malhotra said: 'If all UK diabetics were to follow guidelines reflecting the independent scientific evidence and ignore current low–fat diet government guidelines, it would reduce dependency on diabetes drugs and insulin by over 50 per cent, saving the NHS hundreds of millions of pounds annually.

'Basing diets on starchy foods is misguided and in my view, has been a direct cause of the obesity crisis. For decades, fat has been demonised and led to a huge market in low–fat products, a problem made worse by commercial influence. A complete dietary guidelines overhaul would reverse obesity, type 2 diabetes and heart disease and save billions every year.'

Sir Richard, a former Royal College of Physicians president, added: 'It's more important to cut down on the calories in carbohydrates rather than the calories in fat, because it has caused a tsunami in diabetes. And we are all obsessed by sugar. We need to address this right now.'

However, Dr Alison Tedstone, chief nutritionist at Public Health England, said: 'High–fat diets are often high in calories and can lead to weight gain – this can increase the risk of heart disease, type 2 diabetes and some cancers.

'Too much saturated fat increases blood cholesterol, which also increases the risk of heart disease. We recommend a balanced diet based on starchy high–fibre carbohydrates that are also low in saturated fats.'

The Low Carb Program developed by Diabetes.co.uk has been pivotal in making the case for a change in approach to dietary advice.

In just under two years, the Low Carb Program has a demonstrated cost saving of £835 per person, per year, for each person that completes the program through diabetes medication deprescription alone.

So far more than 270,000 have signed up and taken part in the initiative. Results show that people who complete the program reduce HbA1c by 1.2 per cent (13mmol/mol), lose seven per cent of their body weight on average and one in four people 'reserved' or put their type 2 diabetes into remission.

*15 April 2018*

⇨ The above information is reprinted with kind permission from Diabetes Times. Please visit www.diabetestimes.co.uk for further information.

*© Diabetes Times 2018*

# Should we cut the carbs and opt for fats?

Recent media headlines claim that low-fat diets could increase your risk of early death by almost one quarter. Some media went so far as to question the validity of European dietary guidelines based on the results of a single study. However, the coverage is based on a study that mainly looked at people in lower- and middle- income countries outside Europe. As diets from these countries are considerably different, the results may not be relevant for the general European population.

## The study

This study, published in *The Lancet*, investigated the effect of mainly carbohydrates and fats consumption on the risk of cardiovascular disease and early death.[1] It was carried out in 18 countries around the world, many of which were low and middle–income: three high, 11 medium, and four lower–income countries. Only two European countries were included: Sweden and Poland.

The study was large, looking at more than 135,000 adults aged 35 to 70. At the study start, each participant completed food frequency questionnaires, adapted for each country, to measure food intake. The researchers then calculated the amount of each macronutrient consumed by the participants as a percentage of their total calorie intake. The study participants were divided into groups based on their consumption of fat, carbohydrate and protein, from highest consumption to the lowest.

Participants were followed up after three, six, and nine years to investigate disease rates. After adjusting for age, sex, physical activity, smoking, education level, and waist-to-hip ratio, the risk of death and cardiovascular disease related to diet was assessed.

Out of the 135,000 adults, about 1,600 died from cardiovascular disease and a further 3,800 died from other causes. Concerning individual macronutrients, the researchers found that:

⇨ The people who ate the most carbohydrates (77.2% of total calories) were 28% more likely to die than those eating the least (46.4% of total calories).

⇨ Those who ate more total fat (35.3% of total calories) were 23% less likely to have died than individuals eating the least (10.6% of total calories).

⇨ There was no association between fat or carbohydrate consumption and the risk of major cardiovascular disease.

## Limitations

The study defines a high-fat diet as one including 35% of total calories from fat, which is within the upper-limit of what is recommended by the European Food Safety Authority (EFSA). The media reports that stated that this study contradicts current guidelines are false; the high-fat diet in this study is within the range of current advice in Europe (albeit at the top end).

Similarly, the association between higher carbohydrate consumption and increased risk of death was seen in participants eating more than 60% of daily calories from carbs. This is higher than the current recommendations from EFSA, who advise to get 45-60% of energy from carbs.

The only European countries looked at in the study were Poland and Sweden. Diets in these countries are not representative of all European countries, some will have significantly different dietary patterns (e.g. Mediterranean countries).

Although the analysis was adjusted for some factors, there are many others that were not accounted for. For example, a high-carbohydrate, low-fat diet was linked to the accessibility and affordability of carbohydrates, making them more popular in low-income countries. These are also the countries where other factors such as access to healthcare or poorer working conditions may also have contributed to the risk of early death.

The study only looked at adults aged 35 to 70, who may have different nutritional needs than other groups. A diet lower in carbs and higher in fat may not be as suitable for younger people.

## General recommendations

Dietary fats are important for proper functioning of the body.[2] The fat–soluble vitamins A, D, E and K cannot be absorbed by the body without the help of fats. Some fats (e.g. omega-3 and omega-6) are essential, as the body cannot produce them and therefore need to be obtained through diet. They are needed for vital processes such as brain, eye and heart function, growth and development.3

The European Food Safety Authority (EFSA) recommends a fat intake of between 20% and 35% of total energy intake, while the World Health Organization (WHO) recommends an intake of less than 30% fat. Fat intake in infants can gradually be reduced from 40% of total energy intake in the second half of the first year, to 35–40% in the second and third year of life. This is to account for their specific developmental needs.[4]

Carbohydrates are an important part of a healthy and balanced diet. They can help to control our body weight, especially when combined with exercise. They are also vital for proper gut function and are an essential fuel for the brain and active muscles.[5]

EFSA recommends a carbohydrate intake of 45–60% of total energy intake for both adults and children. This includes carbohydrates from starchy foods, like potatoes and pasta, and simple carbohydrates, like sugars. Eating a variety of carbohydrate foods ensures that we get the maximum nutritional benefit.[4]

References
1 Dehghan et al. Associations of fasts and carbohydrate intake with cardiovascular disease and mortality in 18 countries from five continents (PURE): a prospective cohort study. The Lancet. Published online August 29, 2017.
2 EUFIC (2015) Facts on fats: dietary fats and health
3 EUFIC (2015) 8 facts on fats (Q&A)
4 European Food Safety Authority (2010) EFSA sets European dietary reference values for nutrient intakes
5 EUFIC (2012) Carbohydrates

*6 October 2017*

⇨ The above information is reprinted with kind permission from EUFIC. Please visit www.eufic.org for further information.

# A guide to proteins

*Why do we need protein? How can we be sure we're eating enough of the right kinds? Nuffield Health Nutritional Therapist Tracey Strudwick explains.*

## What is protein?

There are three nutrients that we need in large amounts – proteins, carbohydrates and fats. Proteins in the body are made up of long chains of chemicals called amino acids.

Amino acids can be divided into two groups: non-essential amino acids, which can be made by your body and essential amino acids, which can't be made by your body and must come from your diet.

## Why do we need it?

Proteins are used to develop, grow and maintain just about every part of your body, and they're hard at work all the time:

⇨ Making up the structure of collagen and elastin, found in skin, nails and hair

⇨ Maintaining, repairing and growing tissue, collagen and bone

⇨ Producing hormones, such as insulin, and enzymes that carry out the chemical reactions in the body's cells

⇨ Making antibodies to protect against viruses

⇨ Transporting oxygen around your body in the form of haemoglobin in your blood.

These long chains are constantly being broken down, so your body has to replace them every day.

## How much protein should we eat?

The recommendation for adults is to eat 0.75g of protein per kilogram of bodyweight per day. For a person weighing around 12 stone, that's about 57g/day.

Infants and children, pregnant and breast-feeding women, and people recovering from surgery or injury will need a little more per kilo of bodyweight. This is because their bodies are growing, healing or

manufacturing more cells, and protein is vital in these processes.

You'll also need additional protein in your diet if you want to increase muscle size or you take part in sports such as weightlifting. You can add protein to your diet with a shake as many body-builders do, but most of us get all the protein we need from our food. If you have specific sports-related goals, like building muscle, a professional nutritionist can support you in fuelling your training the best way.

## Where can we find protein in foods?

Fish, meat and dairy contain all nine of the essential amino acids. These animal-derived products are known as 'complete proteins'.

Some proteins, like red meat, are very high in saturated fat, so it's advisable not to eat beef, lamb or pork foods more than twice per week. Try to choose lean meats such as chicken, fish and low-fat dairy products as your primary source of animal-derived protein.

Animal products are protein dense. The list below shows example food types and the grams of protein they contain per 100g.

⇨ Chicken breast (grilled without skin): 32g

⇨ Beef steak (lean, grilled): 31g

⇨ Salmon (grilled): 24.2g

⇨ Eggs: 12.5g

⇨ Cottage cheese: 12.5g

A few plant protein sources contain all nine essential amino acids, and are known as complete proteins: soya beans, quinoa, millet, avocado, spirulina and chlorella. However, most plant proteins contain only some essential amino acids, so they are known as 'incomplete proteins'.

Plant-based products tend to contain fewer grams of protein per 100g than animal products.

⇨ Almonds: 21.1g

⇨ Chickpeas: 8.4g

⇨ Red lentils: 7.6g

⇨ Quinoa: 4.4g

⇨ Brown rice: 2.6g

If you eat animal products, your diet will likely contain plenty of protein, but if you are vegetarian or vegan, eating proteins in combinations will ensure you're getting all of the essential amino acids:

⇨ Whole grains (brown rice, quinoa, whole wheat bread) with pulses – whole wheat tortilla with beans, chickpea curry and brown rice, or quinoa salad with puy lentils

⇨ Pulses (beans, peas, lentils) and dairy products (milk, cheese, yoghurt) – baked beans with grated cheese or lentil dhal with natural yoghurt

⇨ Pulses with seeds and nuts – hummus (chickpeas and pine nuts) or mixed bean salad with flax seed oil dressing

⇨ Dairy with whole grains – cheese sandwich with wholemeal bread or porridge with milk.

Since your body can't store protein, it's best to eat small amounts with every meal or to have a protein-rich snack, to ensure a good supply throughout the day.

*2 March 2017*

⇨ The above information is reprinted with kind permission from Nuffield Health. Please visit www.nuffieldhealth.com for further information.

# The 15 most common questions about healthy eating, answered by a dietitian

*By Tomé Morrissy-Swan*

**W**e humans have become really bad at knowing exactly what to eat to maintain a healthy diet. When once we roamed in search of a healthy balance of fruit, veg and meat, today we scoff a variety of nutritionally questionable but tasty and moreish snacks. Almost certainly, we didn't evolve to eat biscuits and down fizzy drinks all day. But we do it anyway, succumbing to temptation.

Most of us, of course, still know what constitutes an ideal diet. The Mediterranean diet gets plenty of praise, with its focus on an abundance of fruit and veg, olive oil, lots of fish and less meat. Or the varied pre-industrial peasant diet, with healthy grains, veg, potatoes, meat and milk featuring heavily.

It's not rocket science, really. A balanced diet of real food is essential to staying healthy. Yet 50 per cent of food bought by British households is now thought to be 'ultra-processed', increasing risk of cancer as vital nutrients are replaced by harmful additives. Not by coincidence, obesity and diabetes rates continue to rise.

Rather than trying to consume a healthy range of foods, we look for quick fixes – a juice cleanse, perhaps, or intermittent fasting. Evidently, we need help. So we asked registered dietitian Melissa Wilson, who also works for leading dietary food specialists Schär, what the most common questions people came to her with. Here are her answers to those questions.

## 1. How can I tell if I have a food allergy or intolerance?

Reactions to food can involve either the immune system (indicating a food allergy) or no immune involvement (indicting a food intolerance). Symptoms for both vary in type and severity, from immediate to delayed symptoms several hours or even days later. Sometimes allergic food reactions can be severe or life threatening, but in contrast food intolerance symptoms are generally less serious.

If you suspect you might have a food allergy or intolerance it is important to speak to your GP, who will likely refer you to a specialist. Diagnostic tests for food allergies include specific blood and skin prick tests in conjunction with a detailed history taken by a healthcare professional. Whereas diagnosis of food intolerance is by a detailed history taken by an experienced HCP.

## 2. What are the best foods to improve my energy levels?

Having a healthy, well-balanced diet is important to help maintain energy levels as well as eating regular meals supplemented with small between-meal snacks if needed. Starchy foods such as bread, pasta, cereals, rice and potatoes are good sources of energy in the diet, but you should keep the intake of sugary foods to a minimum to help maintain stable energy levels.

The key is to ensure you eat enough for your level of activity (but do not overestimate how active you are). As a rule, for carbohydrates, a portion about the size of your fist is an appropriate mealtime portion and this can be adjusted according to individual activity levels. Around half of our energy intake should come from carbohydrates.

## 3. I am considering going vegan, how can I make sure I am still getting enough of the right nutrients?

A well-planned vegan diet can be healthy and nutritious, but it is important to plan it well to ensure all the required nutrients are included in your diet. Enjoy plenty of green leafy vegetables (e.g. kale and pak choi), as well as pulses, nuts and seeds and different proteins (beans, lentils and chickpeas), to make sure you are getting the right nutrients.

Fortified, plant-based dairy alternatives and wholegrains foods such as oats, rice and cereal-based foods are also important sources of key nutrients in the diet.

## 4. I've heard that fibre is important. What should I eat to boost my fibre intake?

Fibre is an essential nutrient for the normal functioning of the gut and is related to a reduced risk of certain chronic diseases, such as diabetes and cardiovascular disease. Fibre-rich food sources include porridge, high-fibre breakfast cereals, potatoes, wholemeal or wholegrain bread and pasta. A food product is 'high in fibre' if it contains at least 6g of fibre for every 100g of its weight, and is classified as a 'source of fibre' if it contains 3g fibre per 100g.

You can try the following things to increase your fibre intake:

⇨ Having a high-fibre breakfast cereal

⇨ Adding fruit to cereal

⇨ Mixing linseeds with yoghurt

⇨ Choosing wholemeal or wholegrain varieties

⇨ Adding extra vegetables or pulses/lentils to dishes.

## 5. What's the difference between a dietitian, nutritionist and nutritional therapist?

There are some subtle differences between a dietitian, nutritionist and nutritional therapist:

**Dietitians** are the only nutrition professionals that are regulated by law and governed by an ethical code. Dietitians are qualified to a degree-level and use evidence-based research on food, health and disease, which they translate into practical guidance.

**Nutritionists** are qualified to a degree level and provide information about food and healthy eating in a variety of non-clinical roles including public health, health policy, government and NGOs. Only those meeting specific criteria can join the UK Voluntary Register of Nutritionists (UKVRN) and can then call themselves a Registered Nutritionist.

**Nutritional therapists** don't have a degree in nutrition but have an accredited qualification. Nutritional therapists encompass the use of recommendations for diet and lifestyle in order to alleviate or prevent ailments, and the advice they provide may not be recognised as valid treatments by medical and allied health professionals.

### 6. What are probiotics and prebiotics and do I need to eat them?

Natural bacteria in our gut helps us stay healthy, but sometimes the balance of these bacteria is disrupted. Eating probiotics and prebiotics can help maintain this natural balance:

**Probiotics:** 'Good' bacteria can help improve the balance of gut bacteria and can be found in some products such as yoghurts or supplements. Probiotics are generally considered safe for healthy people to consume; however, those whose immune system does not function properly should seek specific advice from a dietitian or doctor before taking these.

**Prebiotics:** Types of carbohydrates that our gut bacteria 'feeds upon'. By eating these, it can help more 'good' gut bacteria to grow in the gut. Natural sources of prebiotics include onions, garlic, asparagus, artichoke and banana.

### 7. I've heard many people are 'going gluten free'. Would I benefit from a gluten-free diet?

Research has shown that although there is no health benefit in going gluten free for healthy individuals, for those with conditions like coeliac disease, a gluten-free diet is the only treatment for the condition.

Some individuals also experience symptoms when eating foods containing gluten, even if they do not have coeliac disease; this is called non-coeliac gluten sensitivity. Symptoms are similar to coeliac disease but it is still not understood how the immune system might be involved and there does not appear to be damage to the lining of the gut as in untreated coeliac disease.

There is a growing body of evidence that a gluten-free diet may help improve symptoms in some people with IBS. Individuals should seek advice from a healthcare professional before making any changes to their diet.

### 8. I do a lot of high-intensity exercise. How can I improve my performance with food?

No matter what sport you enjoy, carbohydrates are the main fuel used by our muscles during high-intensity exercise. Carbohydrate is stored in the muscles as glycogen. Glycogen stores are limited and need topping up each day, particularly if exercising daily or at a high intensity. The higher the intensity of exercise, the faster your glycogen stores will get used up.

You will not benefit greatly from eating carbohydrate during high-intensity exercise lasting less than 60 minutes. However, you can improve your performance by ensuring there is enough fuel in the tank before you begin. The best way to do this is to have a regular meal or snack that is high in carbohydrate two to three hours prior to exercise, such as porridge with milk and fresh fruit or wholegrain toast with poached eggs.

Following exercise, glycogen stores should be replenished with a high-carbohydrate, low-fat snack or meal – you could try Greek yoghurt with berries or a fresh banana smoothie. Refueling is most effective when it takes place within 30 minutes after exercise.

Protein also plays an important role in how the body responds to exercise and is required for building and repairing muscles. The addition of 20–40g of protein to a post–workout meal or snack promotes muscle repair as well as boosting glycogen storage.

Maintaining fluid intake is also critical as dehydration can affect your concentration, strength and power. By consuming adequate food and fluid before, during and after exercise, you can maximise your performance and enhance recovery.

### 9. I suffer from irritable bowel syndrome. What foods should I avoid to help reduce my symptoms?

Irritable Bowel Syndrome (IBS) is a condition that results in a range of gut symptoms including diarrhoea, bloating, abdominal pain and constipation. IBS affects ten to 20% of the population and up to 90% of patients with IBS report various foods as symptom triggers.

In the first instance, simple changes to diet such as having regular meals, eating slowly, and limiting alcoholic, fizzy and caffeine-containing drinks (like tea and coffee) as well as drinking plenty of water, can help lessen the symptoms of IBS.

If the initial advice is not working, a low FODMAP diet may be recommended to help manage IBS symptoms. FODMAPs are a collection of carbohydrates that are poorly digested and absorbed in the gut and can trigger IBS symptoms such as intestinal bloating and pain in some people.

A low-FODMAP diet is a complex three-stage diet and should be followed under the guidance of a FODMAP-trained dietitian. It has been shown to improve symptoms in 70–75 per cent of IBS patients.

### 10. What is the best diet to help me lose weight and keep it off?

Eating a healthy, well-balanced diet is the best way to lose weight and/or maintain a healthy weight, but there is no quick fix. The following tips and lifestyle changes can help:

⇨ Start the day with a healthy breakfast

⇨ Aim to eat three balanced meals per day

⇨ Aim to eat more fruit and vegetables (five portions a day)

⇨ Half fill your plate with vegetables/salad and divide the other half between protein foods (eggs, fish, chicken) and starchy foods (potatoes, rice, pasta, bread)

⇨ Choose low-fat and low-sugar drinks and foods

⇨ Maintain a moderate alcohol intake

⇨ Watch portion sizes

⇨ Avoid eating the same time as doing something else, e.g watching the TV

⇨ Eat slowly and enjoy your foods

⇨ Aim to drink at least 2 litres/day of fluid (water, non–caffeinated/ non-fizzy drinks)

⇨ Include regular physical activity to help achieve weight loss and boost mood

⇨ Set realistic and achievable goals.

## 11. How can I eat a more 'sustainable' diet that is healthy for both the environment and me?

Eating a plant-based or vegan diet has been shown to be beneficial for the environment. It is estimated that a well-planned, plant-based or vegan diet needs about a third of the fertile land, water and energy of a typical meat and dairy diet.

If you are planning to avoid or reduce your intake of animal-based foods, it is important to ensure you maintain sufficient intake of certain nutrients including calcium, omega-3, vitamin D, iodine, vitamin B12, iron, zinc, selenium and protein.

Eating a variety of plant-based foods including beans, nuts, seeds, fruit, vegetables, wholegrains and cereal-based foods will provide all the nutrients required for good health, including essential fats, protein, fibre, vitamins and minerals.

## 12. Can diabetes be treated with diet alone?

Diabetes is a serious, lifelong condition where the blood sugar level is too high. There are two main types of diabetes: Type 1 and Type 2. They are different conditions but are both serious, and can lead to long-term complications if not managed properly.

Type 1 diabetes is an autoimmune disease, and needs to be treated with insulin, but those with Type 2 diabetes may be able to manage the condition with a good diet and exercise alone. However, Type 2 diabetes is progressive and may require medication over time to help manage it.

Nevertheless, a healthy, balanced diet is recommended for all diabetics and individuals should try to avoid sugary drinks to help keep blood sugar levels down. Foods labelled as 'diabetic' or 'suitable for diabetics' are also worth avoiding as they may have a laxative effect and can still have the ability to affect blood sugar levels.

## 13. I have high blood pressure. Can diet help me improve this?

If left untreated, high blood pressure can increase the risk of heart attacks, strokes and cause kidney and eye damage. Making simple changes to your diet can help lower blood pressure, such as cutting down on salt, keeping to the recommended amount of alcohol and eating a diet rich in essential minerals. Reducing your intake of caffeinated drinks may also be beneficial.

It's known that there is a strong link between being overweight and having high blood pressure, especially if the weight is carried around the waist, so losing weight could help.

## 14. How do I need to adapt my diet to make sure I have a healthy pregnancy?

The most important thing is to make sure you are following a healthy, well-balanced diet. However, specific dietary advice for pregnancy includes avoiding alcohol, raw shellfish, raw or undercooked meats, raw or partially cooked eggs, unpasteurised dairy products, supplements containing vitamin A and any dish containing these products.

It is also recommended that pregnant women take two vitamin supplements during pregnancy: folic acid and vitamin D. Folic acid can help prevent the baby developing neural tube defects, so you should try and take a 400mcg folic acid supplement every day before pregnancy (start taking as soon as contraception stops) and continue until week 12 of pregnancy. You can also increase the amount of folate rich sources in the diet, e.g. fortified cereals and green, leafy vegetables.

Vitamin D is also helpful in helping ensure the baby's teeth and bones grow properly and keeps the mother's teeth and bones healthy during pregnancy as well. You should aim to take one 10mcg vitamin D supplement per day all through pregnancy.

## 15. My child is a fussy eater, how can I be sure that she's getting all the nutrients that she needs?

A good diet is important for children as they are growing and developing quickly. However, if your child is refusing food this can be quite challenging! It is important to try to achieve as balanced and varied a diet as possible to ensure an adequate intake of nutrients whilst making mealtimes enjoyable.

Simple tips include:

⇨ Having regular meals or snacks to avoid your child becoming too hungry

⇨ Avoiding distractions at mealtimes and eating together

⇨ Offering small portions on the plate as too much can be off-putting

⇨ Allowing about 30 mins max. for mealtimes to prevent children becoming fed up

⇨ Giving lots of praise if the child eats well

⇨ Making meals colourful

⇨ Offering your child finger foods

⇨ Introducing new foods one at a time.

*17 April 2018*

⇨ The above information is reprinted with kind permission from *The Telegraph*. Please visit www.telegraph.co.uk for further information.

# Eating more fruits and vegetables may prevent millions of premature deaths

By Kate Wighton

A fruit and vegetable intake above five-a-day shows major benefit in reducing the chance of heart attack, stroke, cancer and early death.

This is the finding of new research, led by scientists from Imperial College London, which analysed 95 studies on fruit and vegetable intake.

The team found that although even the recommended five portions of fruit and vegetables a day reduced disease risk, the greatest benefit came from eating 800g a day (roughly equivalent to ten portions – one portion of fruit or vegetables is defined as 80g).

The study, which was a meta-analysis of all available research in populations worldwide, included up to two million people, and assessed up to 43,000 cases of heart disease, 47,000 cases of stroke, 81,000 cases of cardiovascular disease, 112,000 cancer cases and 94,000 deaths.

> "Our results suggest that although five portions of fruit and vegetables is good, ten a day is even better."
>
> – Dr Dagfinn Aune,
> Study author

In the research, which is published in the *International Journal of Epidemiology*, the team estimate approximately 7.8 million premature deaths worldwide could be potentially prevented every year if people ate ten portions, or 800g, of fruit and vegetables a day.

The team also analysed which types of fruit and vegetables provided the greatest protection against disease.

Dr Dagfinn Aune, lead author of the research from the School of Public Health at Imperial explained: 'We wanted to investigate how much fruit and vegetables you need to eat to gain the maximum protection against

disease, and premature death. Our results suggest that although five portions of fruit and vegetables is good, ten a day is even better.'

## Reducing disease risk

The results revealed that even a daily intake of 200g was associated with a 16 per cent reduced risk of heart disease, an 18 per cent reduced risk of stroke and a 13 per cent reduced risk of cardiovascular disease.

This amount, which is equivalent to two and a half portions, was also associated with four per cent reduced cancer risk, and a 15 per cent reduction in the risk of premature death.

Further benefits were observed with higher intakes. Eating up to 800g fruit and vegetables a day – or ten portions – was associated with:

⇨ a 24 per cent reduced risk of heart disease

⇨ a 33 per cent reduced risk of stroke

⇨ a 28 per cent reduced risk of cardiovascular disease

⇨ a 13 per cent reduced risk of total cancer

⇨ and a 31 per cent reduction in dying prematurely.

This risk was calculated in comparison to not eating any fruit and vegetables.

The current UK guidelines are to eat at least five portions or 400g per day. However fewer than one in three UK adults are thought to meet this target.

The team were not able to investigate intakes greater than 800g a day, as this was the high end of the range across studies.

An 80g portion of fruit and vegetables equals approximately one small banana, apple, pear or large mandarin. Three heaped tablespoons of cooked vegetables such as spinach, peas, broccoli or cauliflower count as a portion.

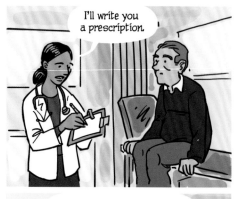

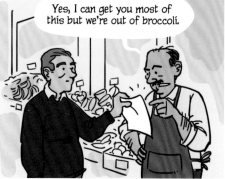

The researchers also examined the types of fruit and vegetables that may reduce the risk of specific diseases.

They found the following fruits and vegetables may help prevent heart disease, stroke, cardiovascular disease and early death: apples and pears, citrus fruits, salads and green leafy vegetables such as spinach, lettuce and chicory, and cruciferous vegetables such as broccoli, cabbage and cauliflower. They also found the following may reduce cancer risk: green vegetables, such as spinach or green beans, yellow vegetables, such as peppers and carrots, and cruciferous vegetables.

Similar associations were observed for raw and cooked vegetables in relation to early death, however, additional studies are needed on specific types of fruits and vegetables and preparation methods. The team say the number of studies was more limited for these analyses, and the possibility that other specific fruits and vegetables may also reduce risk cannot be excluded.

Dr Aune said that several potential mechanisms could explain why fruit and vegetables have such profound health benefits: 'Fruit and vegetables have been shown to reduce cholesterol levels, blood pressure, and to boost the health of our blood vessels and immune system. This may be due to the complex network of nutrients they hold. For instance they contain many antioxidants, which may reduce DNA damage, and lead to a reduction in cancer risk.'

He added that compounds called glucosinolates in cruciferous vegetables, such as broccoli, activate enzymes that may help prevent cancer. Furthermore fruit and vegetables may also have a beneficial effect on the naturally-occurring bacteria in our gut.

The vast array of beneficial compounds cannot be easily replicated in a pill,

he said: 'Most likely it is the whole package of beneficial nutrients you obtain by eating fruits and vegetables that is crucial to health. This is why it is important to eat whole plant foods to get the benefit, instead of taking antioxidant or vitamin supplements (which have not been shown to reduce disease risk).'

In the analysis, the team took into account other factors, such as a person's weight, smoking, physical activity levels, and overall diet, but still found that fruit and vegetables were beneficial.

Dr Aune added: 'We need further research into the effects of specific types of fruits and vegetables and preparation methods of fruit and

vegetables. We also need more research on the relationship between fruit and vegetable intake with causes of death other than cancer and cardiovascular disease. However, it is clear from this work that a high intake of fruit and vegetables hold tremendous health benefits, and we should try to increase their intake in our diet.'

*23 February 2017*

⇨ The above information is reprinted with kind permission from Imperial College London. Please visit www.imperial.ac.uk for further information.

# Do you really need to eat ten portions of fruit and veg a day?

## THE CONVERSATION

*An article from* **The Conversation.**

*Geoff Webb, Senior Lecturer, University of East London*

Only a quarter of UK adults manage to eat the officially recommended five portions of fruit and vegetables a day. In fact, almost half eat less than three a day. It seems unlikely, then, that most people would be able to reach the ten a day suggested by several pieces of research published in the last few years.

Most recently, a paper in the *International Journal of Epidemiology* laid out evidence that upping your intake of fruit and veg to ten portions (800g) a day would further reduce your risk of cancer, cardiovascular disease and premature death. But how strong is this evidence, and how practical is this advice for most individuals or society as a whole? A closer look suggests we need to be cautious about turning this complex research into simple and useful recommendations.

The five-a-day mantra goes back to recommendations from the World Health Organization in 1990 and numerous developed countries have adopted it as official advice. Since then, further research has shown that each of the first five 80g portions of fruit and veg a person eats every day

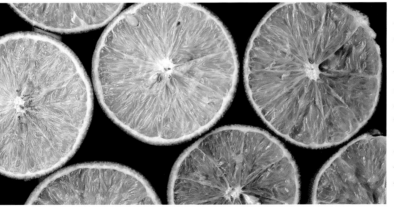

is associated with about a 5% decrease in overall and cardiovascular deaths. But the link between vegetables and disease prevention isn't always that clear. For example, in 2010 the massive European Prospective Investigation into Cancer and Nutrition (EPIC) found

only a small decrease in cancer risk associated with eating fruit and veg.

Then came two studies that have put forward the case for eating even more than five a day. The first, in 2014, linked lifestyle information on 65,000 English adults from the Health Survey for England to mortality records. It reported that the more fruit and veg people ate, the less likely they were to die from cardiovascular disease or cancer. The death rate among those who ate on average under one portion a day was twice that among those who ate more than seven a day.

But fruit and veg intake wasn't the only thing related to the death rate. The one-a-day group were also more likely to be very elderly, male, less well educated, smokers, physically inactive and heavy drinkers. So the researchers analysed the data in a way that took account of these

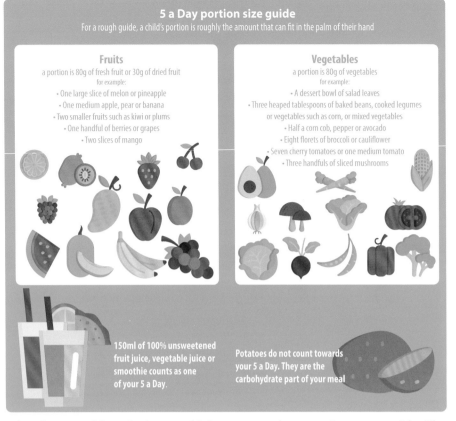

**5 a Day portion size guide**
For a rough guide, a child's portion is roughly the amount that can fit in the palm of their hand

**Fruits**
a portion is 80g of fresh fruit or 30g of dried fruit
for example:
• One large slice of melon or pineapple
• One medium apple, pear or banana
• Two smaller fruits such as kiwi or plums
• One handful of berries or grapes
• Two slices of mango

**Vegetables**
a portion is 80g of vegetables
for example:
• A dessert bowl of salad leaves
• Three heaped tablespoons of baked beans, cooked legumes or vegetables such as corn, or mixed vegetables
• Half a corn cob, pepper or avocado
• Eight florets of broccoli or cauliflower
• Seven cherry tomatoes or one medium tomato
• Three handfuls of sliced mushrooms

150ml of 100% unsweetened fruit juice, vegetable juice or smoothie counts as one of your 5 a Day.

Potatoes do not count towards your 5 a Day. They are the carbohydrate part of your meal

other factors, although they couldn't do this for unrecorded things such as saturated fat intake.

After this correction, the data showed that those who ate three to five portions of fruit and veg were still 25% less likely to die than those in the one-a-day category. Those who ate five to seven portions a day were a further 6% less likely to die and those who ate more than seven a day saw another 3% drop. This meant the biggest benefit was from increasing fruit and veg consumption to up to five a day.

The more recent study brought together the results from 95 cohort studies that each tracked a large group of people over a time. It found a strong association between eating up to ten portions of fruit and veg a day and reduced death – overall, and from cardiovascular disease in particular. But again, the study showed these benefits were biggest as consumption increased up to five a day and were markedly smaller after that. There was also a decline in cancer deaths as people ate more fruit and veg but it was smaller and flattened out earlier.

These studies confirm that increased fruit and veg consumption is associated with fewer deaths, less cardiovascular disease and maybe some decrease in cancer risk. The benefits are particularly seen as people increase their fruit and veg intake up to five portions a day. But the benefits related to eating more than this are much smaller and less certain.

We also don't know for sure whether eating fruit and veg actually causes these apparent benefits. It's possible that they are due to other linked factors or confounding variables, such as eating less saturated fat. Most researchers try to adjust their data to take this into account but there is no statistical magic wand that can do this faultlessly. Some factors are hard to gauge accurately and others might be missed altogether.

However, the association between eating more fruit and veg and living longer is strong, consistent, graded according to how much is eaten and remains strong even after many other factors are taken into account. This means eating more fruit and veg probably does cause the associated health benefits. But we can't say this for eating more than five portions a day. Further studies probably won't change this and nor can they prove cause and effect.

## Weak evidence

The recent studies provide only weak evidence of a small extra benefit of eating more than five portions of fruit and veg a day. We then have to ask whether making this an official recommendation would be worthwhile. For one thing, almost all studies have used middle-aged or elderly adults. So we don't know if ten a day would be appropriate for other groups such as rapidly growing children and adolescents.

What's more, while getting people who eat very little fruit and veg to eat more will likely produce big benefits, raising the official target to ten a day might actually discourage some people. Most people would struggle to eat this much, so failing to hit the target would become expected, and then accepted and excusable.

To get most people in the UK to ten a day would mean the country would have to eat four times as much fruit and veg as it currently does. The environmental, economic and ecological impact of such a massive increase in demand for these bulky products would be enormous and probably unsustainable. Fruit and veg are already expensive in terms of calories per penny and increased demand might make them completely unaffordable for many people. And they couldn't just eat less of other foods because fruit and veg contain relatively low numbers of calories.

Ultimately, these concerns are theoretical because no one expects the bulk of the population to get anywhere near ten a day. But we have to question whether it is responsible to make such recommendations – and on weak evidence – just because you know hardly anyone will implement them.

*14 March 2017*

⇨ The above information is reprinted with kind permission from *The Conversation*. Please visit www.theconversation.com for further information.

# The surprising foods you never realised count as one of your five-a-day

### By Alex Finnis

Do you get your five portions of fruit and veg a day? Remember, the only person you're cheating here is yourself...

Even if you're being honest enough to admit you normally fall short of the recommended amount, you might actually be succeeding without realising, because there are a number of foods that count which you'd never expect.

While claiming fruity drinks like wine and cider count might be pushing it a little, did you know that spaghetti hoops qualify? Great news for five-year-olds and students alike.

Here's a list of foods which sneakily help you towards the magic number:

### Spaghetti hoops

Yes, thanks to the tomato sauce they come in, spaghetti hoops really do count as one of your five a day. A 200g serving will be enough for you to notch one fruit and veg point, so it's time to go and relive your childhood. However, hoops are also quite high in sugar – that 200g serving contains 8g of sugar – so they definitely aren't your best bet if you're trying to be properly healthy.

### Hummus

Chickpeas – the main ingredient in hummus – don't really feel like a vegetable, but they do count as one of your five a day, and what's more, they are high in protein, fibre and vitamins too. Other high-protein pulses like lentils also count, but even if you have a portion of chickpeas and a portion of lentils, that's still only one of your five. Roughly three heaped tablespoons of hummus will sort you out, but if you dip carrots and cucumber in it then you can get a cheeky double win.

### Guacamole

Dip your way to five a day. Yes, guacamole's on the list, and you'll need a similar amount – about three tablespoons, or the equivalent of half an avocado – to make it count. Avocados are high in nutrients and healthy fats, but if you're trying to make guac a healthy option, it's best to make your own, using just avocado, tomato, chilli and garlic, as supermarket-made pots tend to add unhealthy extras. Homemade works out much cheaper, too.

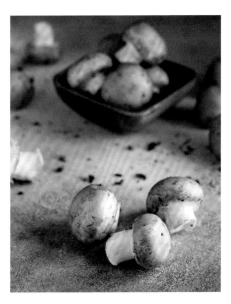

### Sweet potato fries

People always ask whether potatoes count towards your five a day (they don't) but sweet ones do, and eating chips that are actually good for you feels like you're hacking the system, so even better. One small sweet potato's worth of fries/wedges/mash/whatever you fancy doing to them will do the trick here.

### Baked beans

Americans find the concept of us eating beans for breakfast completely bizarre, but while they're pouring syrup all over their bacon like sweet–toothed murderers, we're getting the first of our five a day in bright and early. An 80g serving will do, and beans are also high in protein, carbohydrates, vitamins and minerals, but similarly to spaghetti hoops, it's important to remember they are also high in sugar.

### Onion rings

Half a medium onion counts as one of your five a day, even if you take that onion, cut it into rings, cover them in batter and drop them in the deep fat fryer. It doesn't take us to tell you that this is very much not a good or healthy way to tally up your fruit and veg total, though. You know, because of all the deep frying...

### Olives

Olives are delicious, mostly because they just taste of salt, and salt is delicious. However, they are also high in vitamin E – which you can also get from avocados and kiwis – and therefore count as one of the big five. You'll need to eat quite a lot of them – about 170g worth – so it's best not to rely on olives every day because of the salt content. Save them for an occasional treat.

### Mushrooms

Whether on your breakfast plate, in pasta or even in burger form, mushrooms are on the list if you get three to four heaped tablespoons of them inside you. Mushrooms are also protein-rich, packed with vitamins and a good source of fibre, so as long as you've got over your childhood hatred of them (everyone had that, right?) you're good to go.

### Tomato puree

Don't you just love sitting down and ploughing through a big bowl of tomato puree when you get home from work, just on its own, with a spoon? This is why I was gutted to find out that you only need to eat one-and-a-half tablespoons of the stuff to get one of your five-a-day. That's the equivalent of what you'd put in a spaghetti bolognese. Tomato puree contains antioxidants and is high in vitamins too, so is a great option.

*25 April 2018*

⇨ The above information is reprinted with kind permission from iNews Please visit www.inews.co.uk for further information.

# Food labels

**Nutrition labels can help you choose between products and keep a check on the amount of foods you're eating that are high in fat, salt and added sugars.**

Most pre–packed foods have a nutrition label on the back or side of the packaging.

These labels include information on energy in kilojoules (kJ) and kilocalories (kcal), usually referred to as calories.

They also include information on fat, saturates (saturated fat), carbohydrate, sugars, protein and salt.

All nutrition information is provided per 100 grams and sometimes per portion of the food.

Supermarkets and food manufacturers now highlight the energy, fat, saturated fat, sugars and salt content on the front of the packaging, alongside the reference intake for each of these.

You can use nutrition labels to help you choose a more balanced diet.

For a balanced diet:

⇨ eat at least five portions of a variety of fruit and vegetables every day

⇨ base meals on potatoes, bread, rice, pasta or other starchy carbohydrates – choose wholegrain or higher fibre where possible

⇨ have some dairy or dairy alternatives, such as soya drinks and yoghurts – choose lower–fat and lower–sugar options

⇨ eat some beans, pulses, fish, eggs, meat and other protein – aim for two portions of fish every week, one of which should be oily, such as salmon or mackerel

⇨ choose unsaturated oils and spreads, and eat them in small amounts

⇨ drink plenty of fluids – the Government recommends six to eight cups or glasses a day.

If you're having foods and drinks that are high in fat, salt and sugar, have these less often and in small amounts.

**Try to choose a variety of different foods from the four main food groups.**

Most people in the UK eat and drink too many calories, too much fat, sugar and salt, and not enough fruit, vegetables, oily fish or fibre.

## Nutrition labels on the back or side of packaging

Nutrition labels are often displayed as a panel or grid on the back or side of packaging.

This type of label includes information on energy (kJ/kcal), fat, saturates (saturated fat), carbohydrate, sugars, protein and salt.

It may also provide additional information on certain nutrients, such as fibre. All nutrition information is provided per 100 grams and sometimes per portion.

### How do I know if a food is high in fat, saturated fat, sugar or salt?

There are guidelines to tell you if a food is high in fat, saturated fat, salt, sugar or not.

These are:

Total fat

High: more than 17.5g of fat per 100g

Low: 3g of fat or less per 100g

Saturated fat

High: more than 5g of saturated fat per 100g

Low: 1.5g of saturated fat or less per 100g

Sugars

High: more than 22.5g of total sugars per 100g

Low: 5g of total sugars or less per 100g

Salt

High: more than 1.5g of salt per 100g (or 0.6g sodium)

Low: 0.3g of salt or less per 100g (or 0.1g sodium)

For example, if you're trying to cut down on saturated fat, eat fewer foods that have more than 5g of saturated fat per 100g.

Some nutrition labels on the back or side of packaging also provide information about reference intakes.

## Nutrition labels on the front of packaging

Most of the big supermarkets and many food manufacturers also display nutritional information on the front of pre-packed food.

This is very useful when you want to compare different food products at a glance.

Front-of-pack labels usually give a quick guide to:

⇨ energy

⇨ fat content

⇨ saturated fat content

⇨ sugars content

⇨ salt content.

These labels provide information on the number of grams of fat, saturated fat, sugars and salt, and the amount of energy (in kJ and kcal) in a serving or portion of the food.

But be aware that the manufacturer's idea of a portion may be different from yours.

Some front-of-pack nutrition labels also provide information about reference intakes.

### Reference intakes

Nutrition labels can also provide information on how a particular food or drink product fits into your daily recommended diet.

Reference intakes are guidelines about the approximate amount of particular nutrients and energy required for a healthy diet.

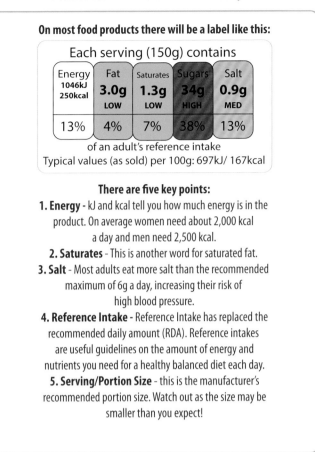

**On most food products there will be a label like this:**

## Each serving (150g) contains

| Energy 1046kJ 250kcal | Fat 3.0g LOW | Saturates 1.3g LOW | Sugars 34g HIGH | Salt 0.9g MED |
|---|---|---|---|---|
| 13% | 4% | 7% | 38% | 13% |

of an adult's reference intake
Typical values (as sold) per 100g: 697kJ/ 167kcal

### There are five key points:

**1. Energy -** kJ and kcal tell you how much energy is in the product. On average women need about 2,000 kcal a day and men need 2,500 kcal.

**2. Saturates -** This is another word for saturated fat.

**3. Salt -** Most adults eat more salt than the recommended maximum of 6g a day, increasing their risk of high blood pressure.

**4. Reference Intake -** Reference Intake has replaced the recommended daily amount (RDA). Reference intakes are useful guidelines on the amount of energy and nutrients you need for a healthy balanced diet each day.

**5. Serving/Portion Size -** this is the manufacturer's recommended portion size. Watch out as the size may be smaller than you expect!

**How do I work out what the labels mean?**

GREEN: Means that the food is LOW in fat, saturated fat, sugar or salt. This will be the healthiest choice

AMBER: Means that the food contains a MEDIUM amount of those listed above. Fine as part of a balanced diet.

RED: Means that the food is HIGH in something, so don't eat too much.

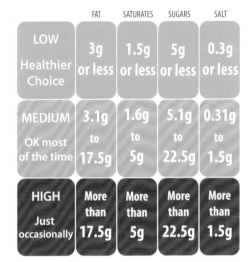

| | FAT | SATURATES | SUGARS | SALT |
|---|---|---|---|---|
| **LOW** Healthier Choice | 3g or less | 1.5g or less | 5g or less | 0.3g or less |
| **MEDIUM** OK most of the time | 3.1g to 17.5g | 1.6g to 5g | 5.1g to 22.5g | 0.31g to 1.5g |
| **HIGH** Just occasionally | More than 17.5g | More than 5g | More than 22.5g | More than 1.5g |

You can use this to help select the healthiest food, remember to choose food with mostly green on the label. Try to avoid food with mostly red as these will be higher than your recommended daily amounts.

## Red, amber and green colour coding

Some front-of-pack nutrition labels use red, amber and green colour coding.

Colour-coded nutritional information tells you at a glance if the food has high, medium or low amounts of fat, saturated fat, sugars and salt:

⇨ red means high

⇨ amber means medium

⇨ green means low.

In short, the more green on the label, the healthier the choice. If you buy a food that has all or mostly green on the label, you know straight away that it's a healthier choice.

Amber means neither high nor low, so you can eat foods with all or mostly amber on the label most of the time.

But any red on the label means the food is high in fat, saturated fat, salt or sugars, and these are the foods we should cut down on.

Try to eat these foods less often and in small amounts.

## Ingredients list

Most pre-packed food products also have a list of ingredients on the packaging or an attached label.

The ingredients list can also help you work out how healthy the product is.

Ingredients are listed in order of weight, so the main ingredients in the packaged food always come first.

That means that if the first few ingredients are high-fat ingredients, such as cream, butter or oil, then the food in question is a high-fat food.

## Food shopping tips

You're standing in the supermarket aisle looking at two similar products, trying to decide which to choose. You want to make the healthier choice, but you're in a hurry.

If you're buying ready meals, check to see if there's a nutrition label on the front of the pack, and then see how your choices stack up when it comes

to the amount of energy, fat, saturated fat, sugars and salt.

If the nutrition labels use colour coding, you'll often find a mixture of red, amber and green.

So when you're choosing between similar products, try to go for more greens and ambers, and fewer reds, if you want to make a healthier choice.

But remember, even healthier ready meals may be higher in fat and energy than the homemade equivalent.

And if you make the meal yourself, you could also save money.

*5 June 2018*

⇨ The above information is reproduced with kind permission from the NHS. Please visit www.nhs.uk for further information.

*© Crown Copyright 2018*

# Vitamins and minerals

*We need vitamins and minerals for our bodies to function properly, and you can find them in lots of different foods. Different vitamins and minerals do different things: for example, some help your body to digest food while others build strong bones. Here, we explain more about these essential nutrients.*

## What are vitamins?

There are two types of vitamins.

**Fat-soluble vitamins** (such as vitamins A, D, E and K). These can be stored by your body but they should also be eaten as part of a healthy diet.

**Water-soluble vitamins** (all other vitamins such as B6, B12, C and folic acid). You can't store these in your body so you need to eat a steady supply from your diet.

## What are minerals and trace elements?

Your body needs small amounts of minerals and trace elements to function properly. They're as essential as vitamins and your body has to get them from the food you eat. For example, you need:

⇨ calcium to make strong bones

⇨ zinc to help your digestive and immune systems to work

⇨ iron to help your body transport oxygen in your blood and to break down and release energy from the food you eat.

### What do vitamins and minerals do?

Vitamins and minerals do different things to keep your body healthy. No one food contains all of them, so you need to make sure you eat a healthy, balanced diet. This means having a good mix of foods to ensure that you get everything you need.

### How much vitamins and minerals do I need?

The amount of vitamins and minerals you need is unique to you. It varies from person to person and can depend on things such as your gender, age, and how much activity you do. There may be times in your life that you need to adapt your diet to suit your changing circumstances. This might be if you get pregnant or as you get older. If you decide to become vegetarian or vegan, you may have to make some changes to your diet to make sure you get all the nutrients you need.

You can also look at the dietary reference values (DRVs) on food labels and supplement packets. These tell you what percentage of the estimated daily amount of nutrients needed is provided by the food or supplement.

### How can I get enough vitamins and minerals?

You should be able to get most of the vitamins and minerals you need by eating a healthy, balanced diet. This includes eating at least five portions of fruit and vegetables each day.

### Storing vegetables

It's best to try and eat vegetables and salad when they're fresh because this is when they'll contain the most vitamins and minerals. The longer you store your veg, the more nutrients they'll lose. Keeping your vegetables and salad in the fridge will help to slow down the loss of nutrients.

Sometimes, frozen vegetables have more nutrients than fresh ones but they also lose them over time.

### Effect of cooking

Water-soluble vitamins are found in fresh fruit and green vegetables. It's best to eat these raw, steamed or grilled rather than boiled because boiling can easily destroy some vitamins and minerals. On the other hand, cooking (but not over-cooking) can increase the amount of, or make more available, some other nutrients. So it's best to eat a variety of food and use a range of cooking methods, as well as eating some raw salad or vegetables.

### What about supplements?

If you eat a healthy, balanced diet, it will usually supply all of the vitamins you need apart from vitamin D. See the section on vitamin D below for more information. You'll usually only need to take supplements if your GP recommends you do so. Here are some examples of when you might need to take supplements:

⇨ if you're planning to have a baby

⇨ if you're at risk of osteoporosis and need vitamin D and calcium

⇨ if you have age-related macular degeneration and need supplements of vitamins C, E, beta carotene, zinc and copper.

Babies and children under the age of four usually need to take some supplements too.

It's important to get advice from a pharmacist or your GP before you take supplements. Some of them (particularly those that contain vitamins A and E or beta carotene) may be harmful if you have too many. They might also interact with some medicines.

Always read the patient information leaflet that comes with your supplements. If you have any questions, ask your pharmacist or GP for advice.

### Vitamin D

Vitamin D is the one vitamin you can't get from your diet alone. It's in foods such as oily fish, but only in small amounts. You get most of your vitamin D from the sun as your body produces it naturally when your skin is exposed to sunlight.

During the spring and summer, you may get enough vitamin D from a healthy diet plus spending a few minutes in sunlight each day. You can expose your legs, forearms and hands to the sun without sunscreen, but remember that too much sun can be dangerous.

During autumn and winter, daylight hours are shorter and it is harder to get sufficient sun exposure for your skin to make enough Vitamin D. Everyone (including pregnant and breast-feeding women) should aim to get ten micrograms of vitamin D each day from their diet. But it can be difficult to get this amount from food, so it's worth considering taking a (ten microgram) vitamin D supplement. There are two main forms of vitamin D – vitamin D3 and vitamin D2. The type produced by your skin is vitamin D3 so check that any supplement you buy contains this type.

Some people can't get enough vitamin D, even in the summer. This might happen to you if you:

⇨ spend lots of time inside – if you live in a care home, for example

⇨ cover up your skin when you're outside – this may be for cultural or religious reasons

⇨ have dark skin – perhaps you have an African, African-Caribbean or South Asian background.

If you can relate to any of these, you should consider taking a daily ten microgram supplement of vitamin D all year round.

Children aged one to four should also have a daily ten microgram vitamin D supplement. Babies up to a year old should have a daily 8.5- to ten-microgram supplement of vitamin D to make sure they get enough. This includes babies who are breastfed and those who are breastfed and part formula fed from when they were born. But if you give your baby more than 500ml of infant formula a day, they won't need to have any more vitamin D. Their formula contains enough for their needs.

Ask your pharmacist or GP for advice if you're unsure.

⇨ The above information is reprinted with kind permission from Bupa. Please visit www.bupa.co.uk/health-information for further information.

| Vitamins & Minerals | Function in Your Body | Food Sources |
|---|---|---|
| Vitamin A | helps you to see in dim light / keeps your skin healthy / strengthens your immune system | liver, oily fish (such as mackerel), carrots, fortified margarine, red peppers, spinach, sweet potatoes, eggs |
| Vitamin D  You can't usually get enough vitamin D from your diet - your body also produces it naturally when your skin is exposed to sunlight | helps you to grow and keeps bones and teeth healthy / helps your body to absorb calcium / helps your immune system work well | oily fish, eggs, liver, fortified breakfast cereals, fortified margarine |
| Vitamin K | involved in blood clotting / builds strong bones | dark green leafy vegetables (such as broccoli and spinach), vegetable oils (particularly soya bean oil), meat, eggs |
| Vitamin B1 (thiamin) | helps break down and release energy from food / maintains muscle tissue / keeps your nerves and muscles working properly | meat (particularly pork), milk, fruit and vegetables, wholegrain bread, fortified breakfast cereals, pulses, nuts |
| Vitamin B2 (riboflavin) | keeps your skin, eyes and nervous system healthy / breaks down and releases energy from food / helps your body to produce steroids and red blood cells / helps your body to absorb iron from the food you eat | milk, eggs, fortified breakfast cereals, liver, oats |
| Vitamin B3 (niacin) | breaks down and releases energy from food / keeps your nervous and digestive system healthy | meat (particularly beef, pork and chicken), fish, wheat and maize flour, milk, yeast extract (such as Marmite or Bovril) |
| Folic acid (folate) | produces red blood cells / in pregnancy, helps to reduce the risk of neural tube defects (such as spina bifida) in your baby | green leafy vegetables (such as kale and spinach), fortified breakfast cereals, chickpeas, most fruits |
| Biotin | breaks down and releases energy from food | meat (particularly liver and kidney), fish, milk and other dairy products, eggs, bananas, vegetables (such as sweet potatoes and spinach), nuts and seeds |
| Vitamin C (ascorbic acid) | helps your body to absorb iron when you eat both together / keep cells and tissues healthy | fresh fruit (particularly citrus fruits), sweet potatoes, peppers |
| Sodium chloride (salt) | regulates fluids in your body / helps your body to digest food / helps your nervous system work well | processed foods, table salt |
| Potassium | helps your body to release energy from food / helps your nervous system and muscles work well / helps your heart work well | vegetables (such as squash, spinach and potatoes), meat (such as beef), fruit (such as bananas and oranges), nuts and seeds |
| Calcium | builds strong bones and teeth / keeps your muscles and nerves working well / involved in blood clotting | milk, cheese, fish, fruit and vegetables, nuts |
| Magnesium | breaks down and releases energy from food / keeps your muscles and nerves working well / regulates your blood pressure / makes bone | green leafy vegetables, nuts and seeds, cereals and grains, milk and yoghurt |
| Iron | helps your body transport oxygen in your blood / breaks down and releases energy from food | meat (particularly offal), fish, eggs, dried fruit, nuts, wholegrains, green leafy vegetables (such as watercress and curly kale) |
| Zinc | produces new cells and enzymes / helps your digestive system and immune system work / repairs tissue / breaks down and releases energy from food | meat (particularly lamb and beef), leafy and root vegetables, seafood (particularly crab), eggs, milk, wholegrains, nuts |
| Copper | produces red and white blood cells / keeps your bones, blood vessels, nerves, immune system and bones healthy | nuts, cereals, meat (such as offal) |
| Manganese | makes and activates enzymes | tea, cereals, vegetables |
| Molybdenum | makes and activates enzymes | meat (such as offal), leafy vegetables and peas, nuts, cereals |
| Selenium | helps your immune system work well / protects cells from damage | Brazil nuts, fish, eggs, meat (such as chicken) |
| Chromium | thought to enhance the action of insulin (insulin helps cells to absorb glucose, which is broken down to release energy) | meat, wholegrain foods, fruits (such as grapes), vegetables (such as broccoli) |
| Iodine | produces thyroid hormone | fish (such as haddock), seaweed, milk and other dairy products, shellfish |
| Phosphorus | builds bones and teeth / breaks down and releases energy from food | dairy products (except butter), cereals, nuts, meat, fish, fruit and vegetables |

# Healthy eating may not offset harmful effects of a high-salt diet

**'An apple a day cannot offset the damage done by eating too much salt in items such as crisps, a study has found,' the Daily Mirror reports.**

Eating a high-salt diet can increase your blood pressure, which in turn increases your risk of serious conditions, such as heart disease and stroke.

In this new study, researchers wanted to see if the risk associated with a high-salt diet was influenced by other vitamins and minerals you can get through general healthy eating, such as eating lots of fresh fruit and vegetables.

The researchers looked at data from the INTERMAP study, an international study of 4,680 people that ran from 1996 to 1999.

They were able to confirm there is indeed an association between how much salt people consume and higher levels of blood pressure.

But they also found that this relationship wasn't affected by what else people ate, such as saturated fat, dietary fibre, vitamins or minerals, and so on.

This doesn't mean there's no point eating healthily if you tend to eat a lot of salt. While you may not 'cancel out' the effect of the salt, eating a diet that's otherwise healthy will bring other health benefits, such as reducing your risk of other long-term conditions.

But better still is to also cut your salt intake. The researchers hope this study will draw more attention to the need to reduce the amount of salt in our diet.

The NHS currently recommends that adults should eat no more than 6g of salt a day – around one teaspoon. Children and babies should have less.

## Where did the story come from?

The study was carried out by a team of researchers from institutions in the US, UK, China and Japan, including Imperial College London and Northwestern University.

It was supported by grants from the National Heart, Lung and Blood Institute, the National Institutes of Health, and by national agencies in China, Japan and the UK.

The study was published in the peer-reviewed journal *Hypertension*.

The UK media's coverage was generally accurate.

## What kind of research was this?

This analysis of the International Study on Macro/Micronutrients and Blood Pressure (INTERMAP) cohort study aimed to better understand the relationship between the intake of salt (sodium chloride) and blood pressure.

It's long been known that consuming more salt is linked to increased blood pressure (hypertension). But previous research hasn't looked at information on what else people ate.

This made it challenging to fully rule out the possibility that other nutrients weren't having an effect (either positive or negative) on the relationship.

Cohort studies like this one are the best way to look at the relationship between what people eat over time and their health.

The main limitation is that factors other than the one being studied (salt intake in this study) can also have an effect on the results.

There are steps researchers can take to reduce these effects, but this may not remove them completely.

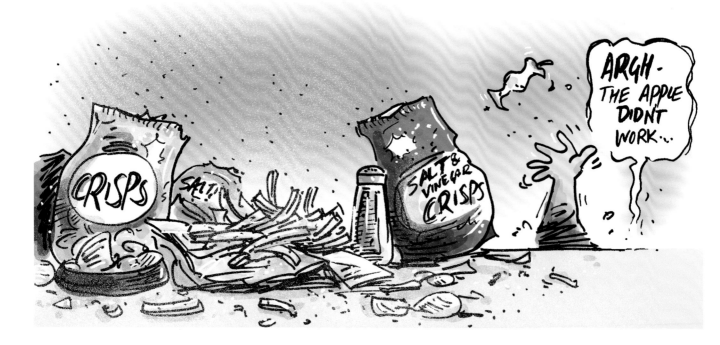

## What did the research involve?

The INTERMAP study involved 4,680 people between the ages of 40 and 59 in the UK, US, Japan and China from 1996 to 1999.

Each participant was required to attend four clinic visits, two on consecutive days and a further two approximately three weeks later.

People were asked about:

⇨ average daily alcohol intake

⇨ if they smoked

⇨ educational level

⇨ physical activity

⇨ adherence to a special diet

⇨ use of dietary supplements

⇨ use of blood pressure medication (antihypertensive) and cholesterol-lowering medication (lipid-lowering drugs)

⇨ family history of cardiovascular diseases and diabetes

⇨ height and weight.

Two timed 24-hour urine samples and detailed data from four 24-hour dietary recalls (all food, drink and supplements consumed in the previous 24 hours) were collected from each participant.

The level of sodium in the urine sample was used as a measure of how much salt was being consumed. The body excretes most of its excess sodium (salt) in urine.

Resting blood pressure was also measured twice at each clinic visit, providing a total of eight measurements of both systolic blood pressure (SBP) and diastolic blood pressure (DBP).

SBP is the pressure exerted when your heart beats and DBP is the pressure in blood vessels between beats.

Participants were excluded from the analysis if they didn't attend all the clinic visits or if any data was missing.

The researchers then analysed this data, looking closely at the relationship between blood pressure and sodium in urine.

They controlled for potential dietary and non-dietary confounders, including:

⇨ age

⇨ sex

⇨ body mass index (BMI)

⇨ ethnicity

⇨ socioeconomic status.

## What were the basic results?

The researchers found people who had higher levels of sodium in their urine had higher blood pressure (both systolic and diastolic).

This was still the case when they took into account the potential influence of 12 nutrients, including saturated and unsaturated fats, sugar, starch, dietary fibre and protein, as well as 12 vitamins, seven minerals and the confounders mentioned above.

## How did the researchers interpret the results?

The researchers concluded: 'The overall INTERMAP data and the US INTERMAP data confirm the adverse relation of dietary [sodium]… show that multiple other dietary factors (macro- and micronutrients), including those influencing [blood pressure] have at most only modest countervailing effects on the [sodium–blood pressure] relationship.'

They advised: 'To prevent and control the ongoing epidemic of prehypertension and hypertension, major reductions are needed in the salt content of the food supply.'

## Conclusion

This study used data from the INTERMAP study to better understand the relationship between salt intake and blood pressure, as well as the potential influence of other dietary factors.

The findings confirm that there's a negative association between urinary sodium and blood pressure: the other macro- and micronutrients analysed didn't have a significant enough influence on the relationship to mitigate the effects of high salt intake.

The researchers hope these findings draw urgent attention to the relationship between salt intake and blood pressure, resulting in a global reduction in how much salt we have in our food.

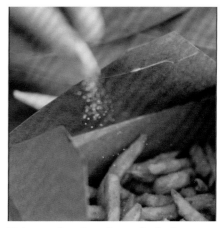

This study aimed to find the true association between salt consumption and blood pressure. But observational studies aren't always able to fully rule out the effect of external confounders on the association between an exposure (salt intake) and an outcome (blood pressure).

The study only looked at the impact of salt consumption and blood pressure in older people aged between 40 and 59. It would be useful to further investigate at exactly what point salt consumption becomes an issue for blood pressure, and whether it has the same effect in younger people.

The INTERMAP study collected data from 1996 to 1999, which is approximately 20 years ago. Salt intake may have changed since then, especially following public health campaigns warning of the dangers of a high-salt diet. Then again, we can't rule out the possibility that salt consumption has actually increased since the 90s.

You can reduce your salt intake by looking at food labelling and avoiding high-salt products, which are marked with a red 'traffic light' warning sign in the UK.

Whether you're eating at home or eating out, don't automatically add salt to your food – taste it first. Many people add salt out of habit, but it's often unnecessary and your food will taste good without it.

*6 March 2018*

⇨ The above information is reproduced with kind permission from the NHS. Please visit www.nhs.uk for further information.

# Healthy vs unhealthy food: the challenges of understanding food choices

**We know a lot about food but little about the food choices that affect the nation's health. Researchers have begun to devise experiments to find out why we choose a chocolate bar over an apple – and whether 'swaps' and 'nudges' are effective.**

The solution to the obesity epidemic is simple: eat less, move more. But take a deep breath before you type these four words into a search engine. The results exceed nine million. Of the top four results, two websites argue against the statement and two for it. Below, arguments about eating and exercise rage fast and furious with dozens of assertions backed by equations, flowcharts, promises of slimming success, and lists of the latest superfoods.

'Despite all we know about food, we know remarkably little about the process of food choice,' says Dr Suzanna Forwood, until recently Research Associate at the Behaviour and Health Research Unit (Cambridge University) and now Lecturer in Psychology at Anglia Ruskin University. 'In a supermarket we're bombarded with the thousands of products on the shelves but most of the time we happily make relatively quick decisions about what to buy. So what's going on in our minds when we reach out for our favourite breakfast cereal?'

When it comes to eating, we're all experts. We're secure in our own opinions (and prejudices) and have no shortage of advice for everyone else. The truth is that, in common with many human activities, our relationship with food is complex and deeply embedded in culture. Forwood says: 'Whenever I give a talk, even to an academic audience, people will listen to me talk about the big picture and then come up to me afterwards to tell me about their personal experiences – typically what they spotted in other people's trolleys the day before.'

We might broadly agree that eating less (and better) and moving more, a message endorsed by the NHS, makes sense – but do we act accordingly? We don't. Finding out exactly what people eat is hard, finding out why they make those choices is harder – and changing those eating patterns is harder still. 'Most of the data we have – and we have lots of it – is observational rather than experimental,' says Forwood. 'There have been relatively few experiments looking at food choice – and those that have been carried out tend to have a low number of participants.'

In the late 1980s government began to realise that it was facing an obesity epidemic on a scale that demanded intervention. Levels of obesity in the UK have tripled since 1980: almost 25% of the adult population is now obese with the UK topping the tables for Western Europe. These worrying figures led to nationwide initiatives to promote healthy living – and increased efforts to understand food choice behaviour.

> *"Perceiving food as tasty is important. It's not good enough simply to tell people what is healthy if they don't think those foods are also tasty."*
>
> **Suzanna Forwood**

Research has shown that obesity is linked to deprivation and low levels of education – as well as to a whole range of life-threatening conditions. Top of the list of 'avoidable diseases' associated with obesity is type 2 diabetes (treatment of type 2 diabetes costs the NHS an estimated £8.8 billion each year), followed by cancer, high blood pressure and heart disease. 'In the past, weight status has long been regarded as a matter of personal choice,' says Forwood. 'And this is reflected by the Government's desire for non-regulatory interventions.' The preference for a light touch approach is exemplified by the establishment of the so-called Nudge Unit (Behavioural Insight Team).

In 2009, the Government launched its Change4Life campaign as a 'movement' to improve the nation's health. Change4Life's online advice for adults makes a series of suggestions for 'swaps' and 'nudges'. Swap a large plate for a smaller one, swap fast eating for slow eating, and swap food high in fat or sugar for healthy fruit and vegetables. Look closely at labelling and make healthy choices based on a comparison of calories and nutritional information.

The current focus is on reducing intake of sugar – not the sugar that occurs naturally in fruit, or even the sugar we sprinkle on our cereal, but the hidden sugar that sweetens so many processed foods and flavours so many popular drinks. In the case of sugar, what is proposed is a financial nudge in the form of a 'sugar tax'. 'Taxes have been shown to be effective but they have to be carefully designed,' says Forwood. 'Sugar taxes, for example, need to avoid raising the price of fruit juices which are high in sugar.'

Do other strands of swaps and nudges work? Research suggests that people are remarkably resilient in their food choices. Taste emerges as the most important factor. Forwood's work shows that healthy foods (such as fruit and vegetables) are not perceived as tasty, particularly by groups who are reluctant to choose healthy foods. She says: 'That might seem tautological but there is strong observational data to suggest that perceiving food as tasty is important. It's not good enough simply to tell people what is healthy if they don't think those foods are also tasty.'

The perception of healthy foods as less tasty than unhealthy foods prompts the question: could product labelling, promoting the tastiness of healthy foods, nudge consumers into making 'better' choices when they're shopping? In research published last year, Forwood and colleagues looked at the 'nudging power' of labelling to increase the percentage of people who might say 'no' to a chocolate bar and 'yes' to an apple as part of a notional meal deal.

In the online study, around half of a representative sample of people expressed a preference for an apple when given the choice of apple

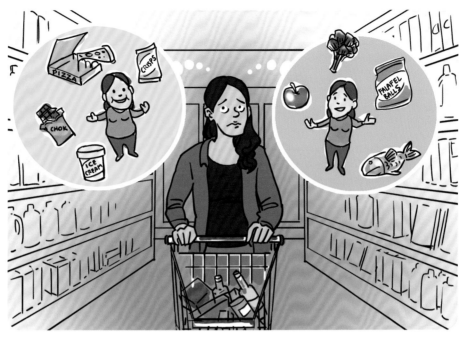

or chocolate bar. Participants were divided into five groups and given the same choice (apple or chocolate bar) with the apple labelled in five different ways: 'apple', 'healthy apple', 'succulent apple', 'healthy and succulent apple', 'succulent and healthy apple'. Labels combining both health and taste descriptors significantly increased the rate of apple selection – to 65.9% in the case of 'healthy and succulent' and 62.4% for 'succulent and healthy'.

Another study, also published last year, looked at the potential for food swaps – often used as part of social media campaigns – as a means for reducing dietary levels of energy, fat, sugar or salt. Using the model of an online supermarket, built as a testing platform, participants were asked to complete a 12-item shopping task. In the course of the purchasing process, they were offered alternatives with lower energy densities (ED). For each item, lower ED alternatives were offered or imposed, either at the point of selection or at the checkout.

'Our study showed that within-category swaps did not reduce the ED of food purchases. Only a minority of swaps were accepted by the consumer and the notional benefits to swaps were slight. It was striking that more

than 47% of the participants offered alternatives did not accept any of the swaps they were offered,' says Forwood. 'Female participants and better-off participants were more likely to accept swaps. This was predictable in that these are the people who we know from other research typically make healthier choices anyway.'

It has been argued that omnipresence of food imagery in the modern built environment, and via all kinds of media, contributes to rising rates of obesity with adverts for less healthier foods identified as a driver for consumption of such foods. A study in Australia showed that people who watched commercial television channels (which carry advertising for fast foods) were, perhaps not surprisingly, more likely to purchase TV dinners.

'What we're talking about here is, of course, observational data,' says Forwood, 'It may, for example, be that people who consume TV dinners are more attracted to certain television programmes that are on commercial channels. Remember that huge sums of money are spent targeting TV adverts in order to make sure that the right population sees them. But this raises the question: could advertising represent an opportunity for policy makers looking to promote consumption of healthier choices?'

'Priming' is described as a psychological effect in which exposure to a stimulus – such as advertising – modifies behaviour. When Forwood and colleagues tested the effectiveness of priming by asking volunteers to look at an advertisement for healthy food (such as fruit) and then choose between healthy and unhealthy, they found that the priming had little difference. The observations were different, however, when the participants were hungry, in which case the preference for the energy-dense foods rose. However, when the hungry volunteers were shown an advertisement for fruit in advance of their choice, the 'hungry factor' was offset by the priming.

The initial experiment was carried out in Cambridge where the participants were predominantly female, well-educated and older – and likely to be in favour of healthy eating. When the experiment was carried out with a more nationally representative sample, the results showed that priming was ineffective in socially disadvantaged groups. 'These people are hard to reach and represent a real challenge to policy-makers,' says Forwood. 'Research tells us that 89% of people want to make dietary changes to improve their health. We need to identify the levers that can support them.'

*11 March 2016*

⇨ The above information is reprinted with kind permission from University of Cambridge. Please visit www.cam.ac.uk for further information.

*© 2018 University of Cambridge*

# 'Junk food' and the consumer blame game

**An article from The Conversation.**

THE CONVERSATION

*Hayley Janssen, PhD candidate, Liverpool John Moores University*

People in the UK are hooked on takeaways and microwave meals, or so we are constantly told by TV chefs and the media. This apparent addiction to fast food is leading to an obesity epidemic.

But what exactly is 'junk food'? And why is the consumer always at fault for failing to resist these hyper-palatable foods?

According to a recent YouGov survey, we eat too much 'junk food' and new research by the Institute of Economic Affairs (IEA) says we can no longer say we do so because it's cheaper. But how can we substantiate these claims unless we agree what classifies as junk food?

With companies such as Deliveroo making it possible to order takeaway food from virtually any type of restaurant, consumers asked the question, 'How many times a week do you have a takeaway?' may inadvertently tell the world they regularly consume junk food. But in fact they may have ordered a takeaway salmon and vegetable dish. And a so-called 'ready meal' containing natural ingredients and little added salt, fat or sugar may face the same judgement.

The IEA focused on this area specifically, claiming ready meals are no cheaper than cooking from scratch – and in many cases they're right. For example, Marks & Spencer's 'Balanced For You' range starts at £4.25 for a meal, which some people may consider expensive for a single portion. However, with an average across the range of less than 400 calories, 10g of fat, 1.5g of salt and 5g of sugar per meal, these ready meals would not fall into most people's idea of junk food.

If we were to agree that the majority of junk food is laden with fat, sugar and salt and that buying healthy food can be cheaper, why do people fail to buy more fruit and vegetables and why do we have such high rates of obesity?

## 'Bliss point'

Studies suggest that genetically we have changed very little since our hunter-gatherer ancestors. We are engineered to seek the most energy-packed food. Despite evolution, we

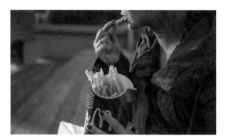

have not evolved at the same pace as our economy or industry – nor our diets. Animal studies have shown that they too favour foods that are high in sugar and fat. The combination of ingredients often referred to as the 'bliss point' is hyper-palatable portions of fat, salt and sugar that are irresistible to our taste buds.

Consumption of junk food often comes down to taste and availability and aggressive marketing exacerbates this. The retail food industry knows that foods high in sugar, fat and salt sell and therefore push such products onto a wide demographic. Advertisements energetically promote these food products. For example, more than 60% of the food and drink adverts during Ant and Dec's Saturday night prime time programme were for so-called junk foods. This did face criticism but it's a regular occurrence.

Even McDonald's, which are supposedly trying to demonstrate 'responsible eating', does so by advertising its apple snacks in children's meals – a not-so-subtle way of promoting fast food to children and their parents. Apple slices, though appealing, do not make the accompanying cheeseburger or chicken nuggets a healthy option.

This isn't solely restricted to the media. It is noticeable in our daily lives, too. As I walk into my local supermarket, I'm immediately faced with a display of 50p jam donuts and hot cross buns and the smell of freshly baked bread. This instantly sets off the hunger hormone 'ghrelin' and makes me want to buy more food as I walk around the aisles.

I counted six aisles with over 100 adverts for high-fat and high-sugar content products. Likewise, almost every end of aisle display boasted promotional offers on crisps, soft drinks, chocolates and other junk foods. The Government advises healthy eating as an easy choice but, as I attempt to bypass the end aisles, I'm bombarded with a wave of promotional signs. In contrast, there are rarely large discounts offered on fruit and vegetables, despite the latest news headline recommendation to eat ten, rather than five, portions a day.

## Advertising and digital media

One global study showed that the most advertised types of food and drink were fast food, sugary cereals and snacks including chocolate and crisps. Therefore, it seems unfair to blame buying habits entirely on the consumer when the majority of these adverts are for unhealthy foods, which we are preconditioned to crave. Digital media also offers another platform for the junk food industry to sink their teeth into. McDonald's has more than 70 million followers on Facebook and KFC has over 45 million. The industry is well aware that peer influence can have lasting effects, especially among adolescents.

For me, the Government is not doing enough to prohibit this kind of publicity in the media and in stores. Theresa May has been criticised for her stance on junk food advertising and blamed for abandoning plans to tackle childhood obesity.

The sugar tax may have some effect as a small number of companies have indicated they will reformulate their products. But is the tax likely to influence consumer choice if it is not coupled with nutritional advice? And where can we get this advice? Our GPs are not trained to explain what constitutes junk food and we have seen NHS funding cuts for child obesity programmes and dietitians.

My research aims to answer some of these dilemmas. I want to discover whether we are actually eating as much junk food as is being suggested. To do this I want to devise a method to help determine people's food intake from urine samples which can assess an individual's nutritional status. If we can answer these questions then we can begin to understand and improve our eating habits and help people with long-term dietary problems.

*25 April 2017*

# Pupils get lesson in healthy eating from pharmacy champions

### Health champions from a local pharmacy visited primary school pupils to help them discover the importance of healthy eating.

Using interactive exercises, staff from Northwood Pharmacy helped Year 1 pupils at Oak Meadow Primary School learn about different food groups, the importance of getting a healthy balance and eating at least five portions of fruit and vegetables a day.

Pupils also took part in a healthy shopping exercise at a virtual supermarket and devised their own food group plates.

The visit formed part of the Healthy Living Pharmacy programme which was launched by the City of Wolverhampton Council, Wolverhampton Local Pharmaceutical Committee and Wolverhampton Clinical Commissioning Group last year.

The quality mark is given to pharmacies which proactively engage with the public to tackle health inequalities and improve well-being, both within the pharmacy and by reaching out to businesses, schools and community groups in their local area.

Carol Haycock, a member of the Local Pharmaceutical Committee, said: 'As a Healthy Living Pharmacy, we believe that every contact counts, and teaching children to look after themselves and respect their bodies at a young age will help them to go on and live well in the future.'

'Children are incredibly good at passing on learning so hopefully they will share what they have learned about healthy eating with their families.

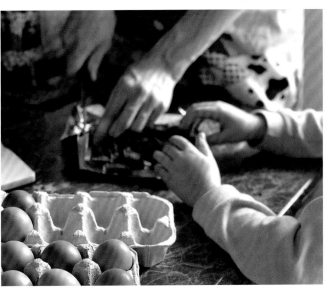

'We hope to build on this in the future and work with other schools and community organisations in the local area.'

Oak Meadow Primary School Headteacher Simon Arnold said: 'In addition to our continual focus upon developing healthy lifestyles, we plan an annual Health Week which provides us with focused time to look at how we can encourage our children to keep themselves safe and healthy.

'The children have enjoyed visits from a dental therapist, the fire brigade and health champions from Northwood Pharmacy who kindly gave up their time to deliver such meaningful workshops about healthy eating to our Year 1 pupils.'

Councillor Lynne Moran, Cabinet Member for Education and Skills, said: 'It was great to see this partnership with Oak Meadow Primary School which enabled the children to identify carbohydrates, fruit and vegetables and protein.

'They know that these foods are healthy and conversely, foods with salt and sugar like chocolate and crisps are best taken in small bites. Such important understanding stands them in good stead for their future health and well-being.'

The initiative also supports one of the central ambitions set out in the City of Wolverhampton Council's Vision for Public Health 2030 – to work with partners and support them to maximise the impact of everything they do to transform health outcome for the people of Wolverhampton.

Councillor Hazel Malcolm, Cabinet Member for Public Health and Wellbeing, said: 'We need to create the right environment for our children to grow up to be fit and healthy, and instilling in them at a young age the importance of healthy eating is a great step on the path to good health and well-being.'

*9 July 2018*

# What are the healthiest foods for a balanced diet?

## By Lowenna Waters

Everyone knows that a balanced diet is essential to enjoying a long, healthy life. And we all know that we're supposed to aim for five servings of fresh fruit and vegetables a day, as well as avoiding the temptations of a McDonald's Big Mac.

However... what does a balanced diet actually mean? Apart from the obvious – a little bit of everything and not too much of anything – it may not be clear what specific foods you should look to eat. For example, it's estimated that 75 per cent of the population doesn't reach the recommended dose of 300mg of magnesium a day. Clearly an imbalance – but how do you fix it?

Fear not – we're here to help. There are a number of nutrient-rich foods that you can add to, or increase in, your diet, en route to attaining your maximum health. Below, we've listed 12 of the key additions, from cruciferous vegetables, to quinoa.

Bon appetit...

### 1. Cruciferous vegetables

Cruciferous vegetables include broccoli, cauliflower, cabbage, Brussels sprouts and kale. They're largely part of the family of brassicaceae, which takes its alternative name crucifare from the Latin for cross, because their four central leaves resemble a cross.

Cruciferous vegetables really have it all: vitamins, fibre, and disease-fighting phytochemicals. A nutrient-packed powerhouse.

### 2. Lean beef and chicken breast

We all need protein in our diets – and for meat eaters, it's beneficial to find the leanest source going. Chicken and certain cuts of beef (ask your butcher) are best.

Studies show that increasing your protein intake to around 30 per cent of your daily calorie intake can reduce late-night snacking resulting in the loss of around half a pound of fat a week. However, you should also be careful not to overeat meat protein –

remember, we're going for a balanced diet here. A few times a week should do nicely.

### 3. Boiled potatoes

Despite falling out of fashion in the post-Atkins era, potatoes are a wonderful, nutritious ingredient. They're particularly high in potassium, a nutrient of which most people are deficient, and which plays an important role in keeping blood pressure at a minimum.

Roasting them is delicious – but also adds unnecessary fat to your diet. Instead, boil them, then allow them to cool for a short while so that they build up resistant starch, a fibre-like substance that has lots of health benefits, including keeping you fuller for longer.

### 4. Quinoa

Quinoa has become an increasingly trendy 'health food' – and the hype is justified. There are multiple health benefits to eating it, including that it's high in protein (a good source for non-meat eaters), anti-oxidants and minerals.

The super-food is often incorrectly referred to as a grain, but it is actually an edible seed that's native to the Andes, and is related to beetroot, Swiss chard and spinach.

### 5. Salmon and oily fish

Oily fish such as salmon, mackerel and herring are a key way of upping your protein and omega 3s – essential to healthy bones, skin and hair. If you are vegan or vegetarian, make sure to include a good quality vegetable-based omega 3 oil to your daily diet, which is abundant in sources such as soy, walnuts, canola oil, and chia, flax, and hemp seeds.

### 6. Beans and legumes

Legumes, a class of vegetables that includes beans, peas and lentils, are among the most versatile and nutritious foods available. They're typically low in fat, contain no cholesterol, and are

high in folate, potassium, iron and magnesium (so there's an answer to that earlier question, for the 75% of people who are deficient). They also contain beneficial fats and soluble and insoluble fibre – perfect for keeping you feeling fuller for longer.

Whip up a bean casserole as a great, protein- and mineral-rich alternative to meat.

### 7. Whole eggs

Eggs are a great source of inexpensive, but still high-quality protein. Eggs are rich in several nutrients that promote the health of the heart, and are recommended to pregnant women as they are rich in choline, which is essential for normal brain development.  As an addition to your day-to-day diet, eggs provide a large dose of vitamin D, which is great for your bones, and prevents osteoporosis.

Why not poach one for breakfast, and eat with some smashed avocado on sourdough? This may sound hipster, but the additional protein will help to keep hunger locked up until lunch!

### 8. Oils, spreads and healthy fats

Oils and spreads are a key aspect in a balanced diet, because including some healthy fats into the diet is essential. It's important to swap cholesterol-inducing trans fats with healthy unsaturated alternatives.

Try cooking with coconut oil, which burns at a much higher heat than other oils, meaning it's less likely to produce carcinogens. Other brilliant oils that are essential to include in a healthy diet are olive oil, and fats from vegetables such as avocados.

### 9. Avocados

Avocados are included in the range of healthy fats – which are essential to the health of our bodies and overall well-being. Some of their many health benefits include that they're mineral rich, they're high in vitamin K which is good for your bones, and they help maintain low cholesterol, which in turn is great for the heart.

Include them in your diet by smashing them on sourdough toast, and eating with poached eggs for a delicious breakfast.

## 10. Nuts

Of course, there are many different nuts, and each has its own specific health benefit. However, as a whole, they're packed with protein, as well as being a source of polyunsaturated fats, and heaps of fibre. A golf-ball sized amount of mixed nuts – about 30g – is recommended as a great mid-morning or mid-afternoon snack.

Almonds are a great source of calcium for those who avoid dairy; Brazils are a source of selenium; and walnuts contain an impressive amount of

antioxidants, which could fight against cancer.

## 11. Fruit and a range of vegetables

Fruit and vegetables are a vital source of vitamins and minerals, and should make up at least a third of your daily diet. It's advised that you aim for eating five portions of fruit and vegetables each day in order to maintain maximum health. There is evidence that people who eat their allotted quota every day decrease their chances of contracting cancer, heart disease and strokes.

## 12. Dairy products or dairy substitutes

There is one main benefit to including dairy in your diet, and that's calcium. Calcium is essential for the normal

development of our bones, and regular consumption is key for avoiding ailments such as osteoporosis in your old age. It's high potassium and magnesium content is also essential for the health of your heart.

If you're avoiding dairy due to a lactose intolerance, it's important to include a calcium supplement in your day-to-day diet. Calcium-enriched alternatives such as fortified soy milk, cheese and yoghurt are great alternatives.

*14 December 2017*

⇨ The above information is reprinted with kind permission from *The Telegraph*. Please visit www.telegraph.co.uk for further information.

# 20 tips to eat well for less

## Can you eat healthily and save money? You bet your bottom dollar you can! Here are 20 tips to help you have your (low-fat) cake and eat it.

If cost is discouraging you from trying to make changes to you and your family's diet then read on: healthy eating doesn't have to cost more.

### Write a shopping list

Draw up a weekly meal plan using up ingredients you already have and make a shopping list of any missing items.

Try not to shop when hungry. People who shop when hungry are more likely to spend more, especially on less healthy foods, such as high-fat and sugary snacks.

### Waste nothing

The average family with children throws away almost £60 of good food every month. Be strict about buying only what you'll actually eat.

Plan your meals so that all ingredients on your list get used. Freeze any unused food. Food storage bags and boxes will come in handy.

### Eat leftovers for lunch

Cook extra portions for your evening meal so that you can have the leftovers for lunch the next day.

Any leftovers can be frozen for another day. Eventually, you'll have a freezer full of homemade ready meals on tap. Find out how to use leftovers safely.

### Buy frozen

Frozen fruit and vegetables are underrated. They come pre-chopped and ready to use, are just as good for you (try to avoid those with added salt, sugar or fat), and are often cheaper than fresh varieties.

Frozen vegetables are picked at the peak of freshness and then frozen to seal in their nutrients. Get tips on freezing and defrosting.

### Try cheaper brands

You could save money by buying cheaper brands than you normally do. There's not always much difference between value and premium ranges. Give it a go and let your taste buds be the judge, not the shiny label.

### Eat more veg

Meat and fish are typically the most expensive food ingredients on a shopping list. How about adding vegetables to meat dishes such as casseroles to make your meals go

further? Or try a few vegetarian meals during the week to keep costs down?

Make it fun by joining the thousands of people who regularly take part in meat-free Monday.

### Cook with pulses

Pulses, such as beans, lentils and peas, are some of the cheapest foods on the supermarket shelf. These pulses are low in calories and fat but packed with fibre, vitamins and minerals and also count towards your five a day.

Use them in dishes to replace some of the chicken or meat, such as a chilli con carne with kidney beans or a chicken curry with chickpeas.

### Freeze leftover bread

Bread is one of the most wasted household foods. Reduce waste by freezing bread, preferably in portions (for convenience) and when it's at its freshest (for taste).

Store bread in an airtight container (such as a freezer bag) to avoid freezer burn.

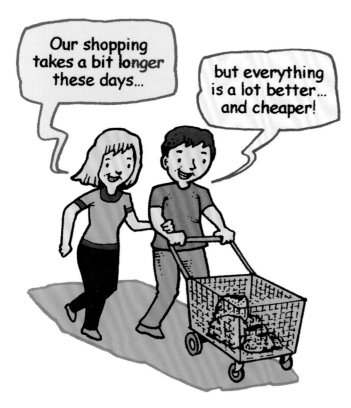

**Our shopping takes a bit longer these days...**

**but everything is a lot better... and cheaper!**

## Know your kitchen

Know what's in your kitchen store cupboard, fridge and freezer. You may find you've got enough ingredients to make a meal!

Plan your week's meals to include ingredients you've already got in and avoid buying items you already have. Check use-by dates to make sure you use up ingredients before they go off.

## Buy cheaper cuts

If you're prepared to take a little more time with your cooking, buying cheaper cuts of meat is a great way to save money. Choosing a cheaper cut of meat, such as braising steak, shin or shoulder, doesn't mean missing out on a tasty meal.

Slow cooking gradually breaks down the fibres in cheaper cuts, giving great taste at a lower cost.

## Look up cheap recipes

Cheap doesn't have to mean less tasty. There are plenty of websites offering recipes for cheap eats and leftover ingredients.

## Eat smaller portions

Try eating smaller portions by saying no to a second helping or using smaller plates. You'll have more left over for lunch the next day and your waistline may benefit, too!

Try weighing or measuring out staples such as pasta and rice when cooking to stay in control of portion size and reduce waste.

## Cook from scratch

Save money by cutting back on takeaways. Preparing and cooking your own meals is generally cheaper than buying a takeaway or a ready meal, and because it's easier to control what goes into your dish, it can be healthier.

## Buy chicken whole

The cheapest way to buy chicken is to buy a whole chicken. From a whole chicken, you'll get two breasts, two thighs, drumsticks and wings, plus a carcass for making stock.

Consider using the deli counter for cheese and cured meats. You can get exact amounts, which is cheaper and less wasteful.

## Compare pre-packed with loose

Fruit and vegetables sometimes cost more pre-packed than loose. Check the price per weight (for example £/kg). Stores know that consumers want to buy in bulk, and so they mix it up: sometimes the packed produce is cheaper, sometimes it's more expensive.

Also, pre-packed isn't always the freshest and you may end up with more than you need.

## Cut down on luxuries

If your regular shopping basket tends to include fizzy drinks, crisps, snack bars, biscuits and cakes, try trimming down on these non-essential items.

Many of these are high in sugar and fat so you'll be doing your waistline as well as your bottom line a favour. They can also contain a lot of salt.

Think about cheaper and healthier alternatives – such as sparkling water and fruit juice instead of cola, or fruit and plain yoghurt.

## Beware of BOGOF offers

Special discounts such as buy-one-get-one-free (BOGOF) deals can offer good value, but be careful: only buy items you actually need and are likely to keep and use – tinned or frozen fruit and veg or rice and pasta are good examples.

Markdowns on perishables at the end of the shopping day are another way to bag a saving – but make sure the item gets used before the use-by-date and doesn't go off sooner than expected.

## Toddlers eat the same

If you've got a toddler in tow, get them used to eating the same meals as you instead of relying on costly pre-prepared toddler food. Simply blend or chop up their portion to suit their age and freeze extra child-sized portions for later. Make sure not to add any salt to their portions and be careful with spicy food.

## Shop online

Price comparison websites, such as mysupermarket.com, let you select a basket of products and then choose the cheapest supplier. The price differences can be significant. Unlike going to the shops yourself, you'll know how much you've spent before going to the till, which can make it easier to stay within budget.

## Shop during the 'happy hour'

Most supermarkets discount fresh items towards the end of the day. However, with longer opening hours it's a case of finding out just the right time to grab those bargains. If you time it right and the 'reduced to clear shelves' can save you big money. Always check use-by dates.

*20 April 2016*

⇨ The above information is reproduced with kind permission from the NHS. Please visit www.nhs.uk for further information.

# Cheap unhealthy food makes healthy food choices much less likely

*By Jack Woodfield*

People are more likely to eat healthier foods such as vegetables when they are closer in price to unhealthier foods, US research reveals.

Scientists from Drexel's Dornsife School of Public Health made this conclusion following an investigation on the effect that price difference has on diet quality in the US.

They examined data from 2,765 people, which was linked to food prices at supermarkets in their neighbourhoods.

The price of groceries was broken down into two groups: healthier and unhealthier. Healthier foods included dairy products, fruit and vegetables, while unhealthy foods included salty snacks, sweets and sugary beverages.

Participants' diet quality was calculated using the Healthy Eating Index–2010 (HEI–2010), developed by the United States Department of Agriculture.

The researchers discovered that, on average, healthier foods were nearly twice as expensive as unhealthy packaged foods, and as the gap between neighbourhood prices increased, participants were more likely to eat unhealthily.

For every 14 per cent increase in the healthy-to-unhealthy price ratio, the odds of participants eating a healthy diet dropped by 24 per cent, even after accounting for factors such as age, sex, income and education.

This impact was particularly strong among people in the middle ranges of income and wealth, and those with higher education.

'We originally expected to find the largest impact among individuals in the lowest wealth/income group. However, given the price gap that we found, healthy food may be too expensive for the lowest socioeconomic status group even at its most affordable,' said co–lead author David Kern, PhD.

Co–lead author Amy Auchincloss, PhD, added: 'Cheap prices of unhealthy foods relative to healthier foods may be contributing to obesity and low-quality diet. We are consuming way too many sugary foods like cookies, candies and pastries, and sugary drinks, like soda and fruit drinks.'

The researchers have stressed the need for policies to be introduced which address large price differences between healthy and unhealthy foods to help improve diet quality in the US and also reduce the risk of health complications such as obesity, prediabetes and type 2 diabetes.

The study was published online in the *International Journal of Environmental Research and Public Health*.

**Editor's note:** Some healthy foods are undeniably expensive compared to unhealthy processed foods, but knowing how to eat healthily on a budget can be pivotal to maximising your health while managing a good intake of healthy foods. Furthermore, it is well worth investing in good health as the payoffs in better health and well-being start early and last a lifetime.

*20 November 2017*

⇨ The above information is reprinted with kind permission from Diabetes Digital Media. Please visit www.diabetes.co.uk for further information.

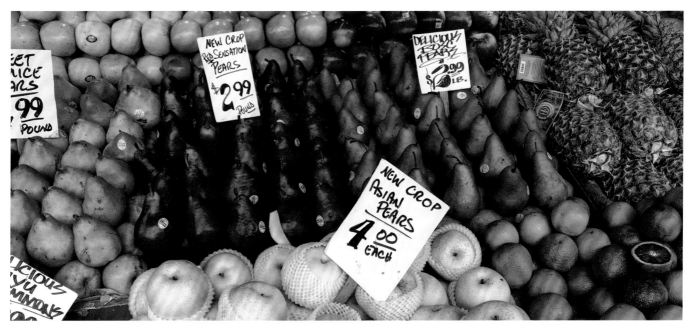

# Food waste and hunger in the UK

**Hundreds of thousands of tonnes of good food is wasted by the UK food industry every year. At the same time, millions of people are struggling to afford to eat. Our work addresses these two issues by redistributing food industry surplus, which would otherwise go to waste, to the people who need it most. Find facts and figures on food waste and hunger in the UK below.**

## 8.4 million people in the UK are struggling to afford to eat

This is equivalent to the entire population of London.

### Hunger in the UK

4.7 million of these people live in severely food-insecure homes. This means that their food intake is greatly reduced and children regularly experience physical sensations of hunger.

UN figures also show that 5.6% of people aged 15 or over struggle to get enough food. A further 4.5% report that they have been a full day without anything to eat.

Our own research shows that 46% of people accessing the services of our charity partners have gone a whole day without a proper meal in the last month.

## 1.9 million tonnes of food is wasted by the food industry every year in the UK

### Food waste in the food industry

By 'food industry' we mean all businesses involved in the supply of food. It includes everyone from farmers and growers to manufacturers and processors to wholesalers, retailers and food service companies.

## 250,000 tonnes of the food that goes to waste each year is still edible

That's enough for 650 million meals.

### Surplus food in the supply chain

We call food that isn't going to be sold, but which is still edible, surplus food. Food becomes surplus for simple

reasons such as over-production, labelling errors or short shelf-life. Surplus food occurs everywhere in the supply chain from field through to fork. Here's a breakdown of where it occurs and how much:

⇨ Farms: 100,000–500,000 tonnes

⇨ Processing and manufacturing: 52,000–160,000 tonnes

⇨ Wholesale and distribution: 80,000–120,000 tonnes

⇨ Retail: 47,000–110,000 tonnes.

### The waste hierarchy calls for food to feed people first

It is a legal requirement for UK companies to operate according to these principles.

### Feed people first

The waste hierarchy sets out five steps for dealing with waste, ranked according to their environmental impact. It states that surplus food should be used to feed people first before it is sent to animal feed or energy.

Currently in the UK, instead of surplus food being used to feed people, many food manufacturers, processors and suppliers dispose of that food via anaerobic digestion (AD) or provide it for animal feed. There are currently a number of government incentives to support AD. While we support this, these same incentives do not exist for feeding people – so we're asking the Government to bring in a level playing field and ensure that it is cheaper for food businesses to redistribute food than to throw it away.

⇨ The above information is reprinted with kind permission from FareShare. Please visit www.fareshare.org.uk for further information.

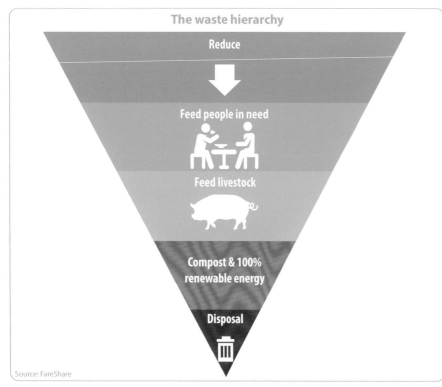

The waste hierarchy

Reduce

Feed people in need

Feed livestock

Compost & 100% renewable energy

Disposal

Source: FareShare

# Save money and reduce food waste with proper meal planning

*By Hayley Mitchell*

We've all been there. You've just been food shopping, the cupboards are stocked, yet you haven't a clue what to cook for dinner. A house full of food but not a meal in sight! Or, maybe you're stuck because you have a full day of work and no time to go to the shops.

Some clever meal planning can help ensure you only buy what you need. Saving not only money, but on food waste too.

## Meal planning is…

### Organised

Meal planning is asking the 'what do want for dinner?' question a week in advance. It's deciding your meals for the week and buying all the necessary ingredients in one shop.

It's also preparing ingredients in advance as much as possible. Then you won't have the, 'I can't face peeling those now, I'm starving' dilemmas.

### Money saving

Planning your meals for the week means no unnecessary supermarket purchases. Scouring the shops looking for inspiration and picking random ingredients can end up producing waste. Write a list of the ingredients you need to buy and stick to it! You'll build up a good basic store cupboard, and will only need to buy a few fresh items for each meal.

If you're keen to save even more money and time on meals, it may be worth investing in a pressure cooker too.

### Healthier eating

If you're trying to eat healthily, meal planning is ideal. Planning in advance avoids last-minute, ready meals and helps you to resist temptation.

Also, if you are following a specific diet (for example if you've been diagnosed with an allergy), it can take time to get used to a new way of eating. A little forethought helps ensure you stick to your plan.

### Less wasteful

Planning meals in advance and only buying what you need means wasting less.

Food waste is a huge problem, with the UK binning approximately £13-billion- worth of food in 2015. Not only will you save money, stress and eat healthier. You'll also have the satisfaction of knowing you're being less wasteful.

It's also a good idea to plan a 'leftovers' night into your schedule too. That way you really will minimise food waste. Find out more about how you can turn forgotten veg into tasty treats.

## How do I get started with meal planning?

### Set a schedule

The first step to meal planning is to decide when your week will run from. For me a Sunday night is the ideal time to sit down, plan meals and write a thorough shopping list. This means that on a Monday I can order my shopping to be delivered for the week. Monday's meal is usually something quick and easy, as I know I won't be able to prep the night before.

Choose a schedule that fits with your routine and you're more likely to stick to it. If you tend to do a grocery shop at the weekend, do your meal planning on a Friday.

At this point, also consider what your weekly schedule is like. What nights do you work late? Plan a slow cooker meal or something quick and easy to make here. When do you tend to need a comfort meal? Is it at the start of the working week to get you through? Do you like a treat or take out on a Friday? Account for these when you're meal planning so that you have meals that suit your needs. Being stuck with something you don't fancy when the time comes is really uninspiring.

### Get planning

Now find yourself a planning format that works for you. There are loads of templates available. We love using printable meal planners. They come with a variety of different styles to suit your needs.

Templates can include all three meals for the day or just your main meal. Several also include a shopping list section to get you organised. Others even include space to reflect on what did and didn't work to help with future planning.

### Shop for what you need

For me, meal planning works really well with online shopping. You can sit at a computer with your shopping list to hand and order exactly what you need. Free from the temptation of wandering the aisles on an empty stomach!

You can even use meal planning apps which mean your shopping list can be online. Some paid-for apps will transfer your list directly to your online shopping basket.

### Prep and enjoy

Meal planning works well if you prepare the day before. It saves stress, and time that could be spent at the table. You could even prepare most of your meals at the start of the week, leaving very little to do but heat them up each night.

Then, you can sit back and enjoy healthy, cost-efficient meals every night of the week!

⇨ The above information is reprinted with kind permission from The Food Rush. Please visit www.thefoodrush.com for further information.

*©The Food Rush 2018*

# Key facts

- Worldwide obesity has nearly tripled since 1975. (page 1)

- Over 340 million children and adolescents aged five to 19 were overweight or obese in 2016. (page 1)

- While just under 1% of children and adolescents aged five to 19 were obese in 1975, more 124 million children and adolescents (6% of girls and 8% of boys) were obese in 2016. (page 1)

- Childhood obesity is associated with a higher chance of obesity, premature death and disability in adulthood. (page 2)

- The UK is the most overweight nation in Western Europe, with levels of obesity growing faster than in the US. (page 3)

- Tax on drinks with more than five grams of sugar per 100ml will be levied by 18p per litre, while those with eight grams or more of sugar per 100ml will have an extra tax of 24p per litre. (page 3)

- Being overweight or obese as an adult is linked to 13 different types of cancer including breast, bowel and kidney cancer, but only 15% of people in the UK are aware of the link. (page 4)

- 'Verbal pushes' meant 34 per cent of customers ended up buying a larger coffee than requested, with 33 per cent upgrading to meal deals, and 36 per cent adding chocolate to their shop. (page 5)

- Young people aged 18 to 24 are the most likely to experience up-selling, with the study finding that they consume an extra 750 calories a week as a result, which could mean an annual gain of up to 11 pounds. (page 5)

- In England, an estimated 16% of children aged two to 15 were obese in 2016, and a further 12% were overweight (but not obese). That means 28% of two to 15 year olds were overweight or obese – so just over a quarter. (page 6)

- 29% of girls were estimated to be overweight or obese, and 26% of boys were. (page 6)

- In Wales, an estimated 27% of children aged four to five were overweight or obese in 2016/17, based on the Childhood Measurement Programme for Wales. (page 6)

- In Scotland, an estimated 23% of four- to five-year-olds were 'at risk' of being overweight or obese in 2016/17. (page 6)

- 3.7 million children in the UK are living in these households, earning less than £15,860, and are likely to be unable to afford a healthy diet as defined by the Government. (page 13)

- Over a quarter (26%) of Year 6 children in the most deprived areas of England are obese, but obesity affects just 11% in England's richest communities – and the gap is growing. (page 13)

- Out of the 135,000 adults, about 1,600 died from cardiovascular disease and a further 3,800 died from other causes. (page 15)

- The people who ate the most carbohydrates (77.2% of total calories) were 28% more likely to die than those eating the least (46.4% of total calories). (page 15)

- The European Food Safety Authority (EFSA) recommends a fat intake of between 20% and 35% of total energy intake, while the World Health Organization (WHO) recommends an intake of less than 30% fat. (page 15)

- 50 per cent of food bought by British households is now thought to be 'ultra-processed'. (page 17)

- IBS affects ten to 20% of the population and up to 90% of patients with IBS report various foods as symptoms triggers. (page 18)

- Fruit and vegetable intake above five-a-day shows major benefit in reducing the chance of heart attack, stroke, cancer and early death. (page 20)

- Approximately 7.8 million premature deaths worldwide could be potentially prevented every year if people ate ten portions, or 800g, of fruit and vegetables a day. (page 20)

- Even a daily intake of 200g was associated with a 16 per cent reduced risk of heart disease, an 18 per cent reduced risk of stroke and a 13 per cent reduced risk of cardiovascular disease. (page 20)

- Only a quarter of UK adults manage to eat the officially recommended five portions of fruit and vegetables a day. (page 21)

- The one-a-day group were also more likely to be very elderly, male, less well educated, smokers, physically inactive and heavy drinkers. (page 21)

- Those who ate three to five portions of fruit and veg were still 25% less likely to die than those in the one-a-day category. (page 22)

- Most people in the UK eat and drink too many calories, too much fat, sugar and salt, and not enough fruit, vegetables, oily fish or fibre. (page 24)

- Eating a high-salt diet can increase your blood pressure, which in turn increases your risk of serious conditions, such as heart disease and stroke. (page 28)

- It's estimated that 75 per cent of the population doesn't reach the recommended dose of 300mg of magnesium a day. (page 34)

- 8.4 million people in the UK are struggling to afford to eat. (page 38)

- UN figures also show that 5.6% of people aged 15 or over struggle to get enough food. (page 38)

- 1.9 million tonnes of food is wasted by the food industry every year in the UK. (page 38)

- 250,000 tonnes of the food that goes to waste each year is still edible. (page 38

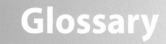

### BMI (body mass index)

An abbreviation which stands for 'body mass index' and is used to determine whether an individual's weight is in proportion to their height. If a person's BMI is below 18.5 they are usually seen as being underweight. If a person has a BMI greater than or equal to 25, they are classed as overweight and a BMI of 30 and over is obese. As BMI is the same for both sexes and adults of all ages, it provides the most useful population-level measure of overweight and obesity. However, it should be considered a rough guide because it may not correspond to the same degree of 'fatness' in different individuals (e.g. a body builder could have a BMI of 30 but would not be obese because his weight would be primarily muscle rather than fat).

### Diet

The variety of food and drink that someone eats on a regular basis. The phrase 'on a diet' is also often used to refer to a period of controlling what one eats while trying to lose weight.

### Eatwell Guide

The Eatwell Guide has replaced the Eatwell plate. It shows the different types of food we need to eat – and in what proportions – to have a well-balanced and healthy diet. Based on the eatwell guide, people should try to eat: plenty of fruit and vegetables; plenty of potatoes, bread, rice, pasta and other starchy foods; some milk and dairy foods; some meat, fish, eggs, beans and other non-dairy sources of protein; and just a small amount of foods and drinks that are high in fat or sugar.

### Fat

Fat is an essential part of our diet. Our bodies require small amounts of 'good fat' to function and help prevent disease. However, too much fat, especially of the wrong type, can cause serious health problems such as obesity, higher blood pressure and cholesterol levels, which in turn lead to a greater risk of heart disease. The two main types of fat are saturated and unsaturated. Unsaturated fats (e.g. found in oily fish) are generally considered better for us than saturated fats (such as dairy products, like cheese).

### Food poverty

When people struggle to afford food. The UK has seen an increase in the use of food banks and food parcels. The Trussel Trust food bank use remains at a record high with over one million three-day emergency food supplies given to people in crisis in 2015/16.

### Food waste

Around seven million tonnes of food is thrown away by households in the UK every year. Some of the waste is unavoidable, such as peelings or bones, but most of the food is edible. This is because there is often confusion over use-by and best-before dates. Also many families buy more food than they actually need.

### Junk food

'Junk' food is a widely-used term for unhealthy and fatty food with little nutritional value. It is usually associated with 'fast' or takeaway food.

### Nutrition

The provision of materials needed by the body for growth, maintenance and sustaining life. Commonly when people talk about nutrition, they are referring to the healthy and balanced diet we all need to eat in order for the body to function properly.

### Obesity

When someone is overweight to the extent that their BMI is 30 or above, they are classed as obese. Obesity is increasing in the UK and is associated with a number of health problems, such as an increased risk of heart disease and type 2 diabetes. Worldwide obesity has more than doubled since 1980 and this is most likely due to our more sedentary lifestyle, combined with a lack of physical exercise.

### Protein

Proteins are chains of amino acids that allow the body to build and repair body tissue. Protein is found in dairy foods, meat, fish and soya beans.

### Starch

Starch is a complex carbohydrate found in potatoes, rice, corn, wheat and other foods. It is made up of glucose and allows animals and plants to store energy as fat.

### Sugar

Sugar is a carbohydrate that is a naturally-occurring nutrient that makes food taste sweet. There are a number of different sugars: glucose and fructose are found in fruit and vegetables; milk sugar is known as lactose; maltose (malt sugar) is found in malted drinks and beer; and sucrose comes from sugar cane or beet and is often referred to as 'table' or 'added' sugar. It also occurs naturally in some fruit and vegetables.

### Sweeteners

Artificial sweeteners are low-calorie/calorie-free chemical substances used instead of sugar. They are found in thousands of products, such as drinks, desserts, ready meals and even toothpaste. There is much debate on the potential toxic side effects of consuming sweeteners.

### Traffic light labelling

A new food labelling system, implemented by large food manufacturers and supermarkets to provide clear nutritional information to their consumers. Red, amber and green labels are used on food packaging to indicate how healthy that food is considered, with a green label indicating a very healthy food and red indicating a food that is high in salt, sugar or fats and which should therefore be enjoyed only in moderation.

### Vitamins

Organic compounds that are essential to the body, but only in very small quantities. Most of the vitamins and minerals we need are provided through a balanced diet: however, some people choose to take additional vitamin supplements.

# Assignments

## Brainstorming

⇨ In small groups, discuss what you know about food and diet. Consider the following points:

- What is the Eatwell Guide?

- What is food poverty?

- What is food waste? How can it be avoided?

⇨ What is body mass index (BMI) and how is it used to measure whether someone is a healthy weight? Is it a useful tool? Can you think of any problems with the way BMI is calculated?

## Research

⇨ How many cookery and food-related programmes are shown on television in the course of a week? Do any of these programmes explore healthy eating? Over the course of a week, make a note of all the food-related programmes you come across. Share your findings with your class and discuss why you think cooking/food programmes are popular, and whether they encourage or discourage healthy eating.

⇨ How much food do you throw away? Over the course of seven days, keep track of how much food waste your household produces. How could this food waste have been avoided? Write a report analysing your findings and include suggestions for how you might reduce your household food waste in future.

⇨ How much does your family spend on an average food shop per week? Make some notes on how you think you could reduce the cost of the food shopping, whilst ensuring that you are eating a balanced diet. Compare the amounts your families spend with your class.

⇨ Do you eat your 5-a-Day? Over the course of one week, make a note of how many portions of fruit and vegetables you eat. Have you eaten more or less than you thought? Make some notes and discuss with your class.

## Design

⇨ Design a leaflet explaining food poverty in Britain. You should describe what food banks and food parcels are. You might also want to include details about organisations people can turn to if they are experiencing difficulties, such as information about the Trussell Trust.

⇨ Create a poster that clearly explains the traffic light colour-coded food labels.

⇨ Create your own cookbook which includes recipes on the theme of 'eating healthy on a budget'. Think of a name for your cookbook and include at least three original recipes.

⇨ Design an informative leaflet about the importance of vitamins and minerals. Use the article 'Vitamins and minerals' on page 26.

⇨ Choose a country in Europe and research their relationship with food. How does it differ from the situation in the UK? What foods are traditionally eaten? Create a PowerPoint or Prezi presentation that compares and contrasts your chosen country's food and diet with those of the UK.

⇨ Choose one of the articles from this book and create your own illustration that highlights the key themes of the text.

## Oral

⇨ With a partner, role-play a radio interview on the topic of 'the sugar tax'. The interviewee, a campaigner for health charity, should give advice on how sugar effects the body. The interviewer should ask questions for and against the tax.

⇨ Choose one of the illustrations from this book and, with a partner, discuss what you think the artist was trying to portray.

⇨ With a partner, discuss what an ideal, balanced meal would be based on the Eatwell Guide, use the article 'Eating a balanced diet', on page 11.

⇨ In small groups, discuss how you could add more fruit and vegetables to your school menu. Do you think that there is enough already? Would you like more? Make some notes and present to the rest of your class.

## Reading/writing

⇨ Read 'Junk Food' and the consumer blame game on page 32. Write a letter to a supermarket to persuade them to reduce the amount of junk food that is available.

⇨ Read 'How the war changed nutrition: from there to now' on page 9. Write a short essay exploring how food and diet has changed over time. You might want to look at the ways in which food and diet have been affected by modern conveniences.

⇨ Write a letter to your head teacher explaining why you believe it is important for students to be taught about diet and nutrition at school.

⇨ Read through some newspapers or magazines. How many articles are about food? Are there any recipes?

⇨ Create a meal plan for one day and write a paragraph why you think that this is a good or bad plan. Is it balanced? Write another paragraph on how you could improve the plan.

# Acknowledgements

The publisher is grateful for permission to reproduce the material in this book. While every care has been taken to trace and acknowledge copyright, the publisher tenders its apology for any accidental infringement or where copyright has proved untraceable. The publisher would be pleased to come to a suitable arrangement in any such case with the rightful owner.

## Images

All images courtesy of iStock except pages 5, 12, 13, 23, 25, 31, 37: Unsplash. 8, 10, 21, 32, 35: Pixabay.

## Icons

Icons on pages 12, 22 and 38 were made by Freepik from www.flaticon.com.

Icons on page 12 were made by Smashicons from www.flaticon.com.

## Illustrations

Don Hatcher: pages 4 & 36. Simon Kneebone: pages 10 & 28. Angelo Madrid: pages 20 & 31.

## Additional Acknowledgements

Page 1: World Heath Organization, 2018, Obesity and overweight, Available at <www.who.int/news-room/fact-sheets/detail/obesity-and-overweight> [Accessed 1 August 2018]

Page 4: Cancer Research UK, https://www.cancerresearchuk.org/about-us/cancer-news/press-release/2018-02-26-millennials-top-obesity-chart-before-reaching-middle-age [Accessed 1 August 2018]

With thanks to the Independence team: Shelley Baldry, Danielle Lobban, Jackie Staines and Jan Sunderland.

Tina Brand

Cambridge, October 2018